Karen & Jaime

Life and Love are the greatest gifts we can give one another. Each day should be filled with Kindness, joy, love, gratitude, forgiveness and services to others.

Janice Herring

Meaghan's Story
More Than Just A Statistic

ALL RIGHTS RESERVED -- No part of this book may be reproduced in any form or by any electronic or mechanical means including information storage and retrieval systems without permission in writing from the author or the publisher.

Copyright © 2010 - Janice Herrity and Deeds Publishing
Printed in the United States of America

Cover photo courtesy of Flashes of Hope
Other photos are from the author's private collection
Facts on cancer are from http://www.curesearch.org,
http://www.alexslemonade.org/resources/facts,
http://www.kristinasrainbowsofhope.org/facts.html,
http://www.morganadamsfoundation.org/statistics.html, and
http://www.danisfoundation.org/?page=PediatricCancerStatistics

Published by Deeds Publishing, Marietta, GA

First Edition, September 2010

For information write Deeds Publishing, PO Box 682212, Marietta, GA 30068 or www.deedspublishing.com

ISBN 978-0-9826180-4-2

Meaghan's Story
More Than Just A Statistic

Janice Herrity

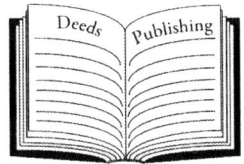

Acknowledgement

I wrote this book as a promise to my daughter, Meaghan, and would have never finished it without the support of my husband, Jim, and sons, Jimmy and TJ. I thank the many friends who read my rough drafts and encouraged me throughout my two year endeavor with positive feedback and assured me that Meaghan's Story needed to be told.

Special thanks to Julia Mulherin and Kim Clore who never left my side during Meaghan's illness. They packed our old house, coordinated the move, prepared the house for sale, arranged our new home, organized meals, spent the night so I could get a few hours sleep, listened to me vent, and wept alongside our family.

I also need to thank Jessica Bailey and Erin Duzan-Hachey, Meaghan's cousins. These young women stepped forward to assist us out of love of family. They became the sisters Meaghan never had but had always wished for. I am eternally grateful to both for the hours they spent with Meaghan when she was at her lowest point emotionally, for helping to rebuild her confidence, and for providing hours of laughter and love.

I also want to thank the many wonderful charitable organizations that helped us during Meaghan's illness. Edmarc Hospice for Children, Make A Wish Foundation, and Flashes of Hope each made our journey a little easier. There are no words to express my gratitude to the doctors, nurses, therapists, and social workers at CHKD and Edmarc. They always treated Meaghan with dignity and respect, they valued her opinion, and they helped her mature through the adversity. Each day, I continue to marvel at the work that they do. These dedicated medical professional are truly angels among us.

I need to thank Meaghan's friends who were a constant in her life and never left her side. Meaghan's greatest fear was that she would be abandoned because of her illness, but fortunately this never became an issue. Thank you to Katie Andleton, Krystin Rizzo, Taylor Huskey, Charlie Barnett, Shelby Decker, Laura Buckley, and Melissa Chromik for your gifts of friendship and laughter. Your friendship helped Meaghan through some of the toughest days of her life.

Thank you to Coaches Don Samuels and Phil Sheldon for your support, encouraging words, and friendship – it meant the world to both Meaghan and our family. Thank you to Amy Moore for reading my manuscript and passing it along to Bob Babcock, president of Deeds Publishing. This book would never have been published without you.

Thank you to our family pediatrician, Dr. David Holzsager, who was a constant ally and presence during Meaghan's illness. Thank you to my sister, Karen; your strength, grace, faith, and advice were invaluable. You provided the roadmap Meaghan and I followed as we navigated the world of terminal illness.

Lastly, to Meaghan: you taught me more about life, love, and courage then I could have ever taught you. Thank you for watching us from above. We continue to feel your presence, and you have taught us that life and love do not end with death.

Dedication

To Meaghan,

Your strength, courage, and quiet grace through adversity continue to inspire us daily.

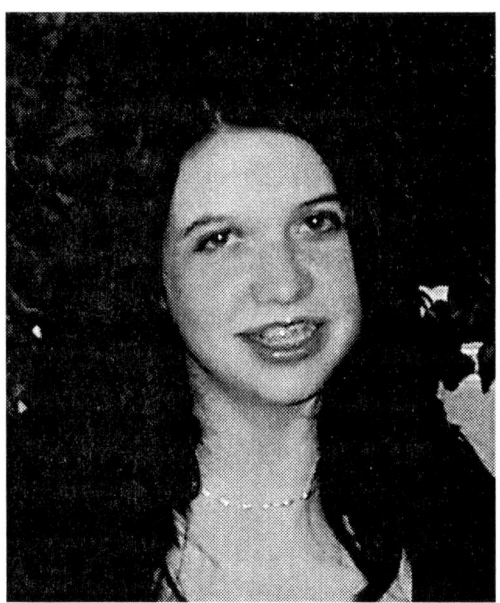

From Meaghan's Friends and Family

I am still in shock that this happened to my dear friend. Meaghan was so brave and never once complained. I can only hope to have half as much poise and grace as she did. I am so honored to call her my friend and I miss her every day.

Krystin Rizzo (Dear friend of Meaghan's)

I've always believed in God and life after death, but being with Meaghan for the last few days of her life strengthened my faith. During this time, Meaghan drifted between our world and the afterlife. She told us about walking on the beach with her grandfather, Papa, his wacky wardrobe, her need for new flip flops, and the sights and sounds of what she was experiencing. Since Meaghan could no longer walk, I knew that she was crossing over and experiencing what it would be like on the "other side". What a special gift she had given me that day! Don't sweat the small stuff, tell your family you love them, and live a good life because there is definitely a Heaven when you leave Earth.

Kim Clore (Friend of Janice)

Meaghan Herrity was an exceptional student. She was also an exceptional teacher. She taught us how to live with hope and optimism. She taught us how to laugh with microwave peeps and sling shot monkeys. She taught us how to love – unconditionally and with forgiveness and she taught us how to die – with grace and dignity.

Kathy Eanes (Meaghan's teacher and friend of family)

Although I was only able to spend mere years with her, Meags has made a greater impact on my life than any person I have, or will know. It only makes sense to tell her unbelievable story to as many as we can. Her life deserves to be celebrated and revered.

Katie Andelton (Meaghan's best friend)

Although my friendship with Meaghan coincided with the toughest two years of her life and mine, the time we spent together was filled with laughter.

Taylor Huskey (dear friend of Meaghan's)

Meaghan was truly an inspiration to me, she has left an everlasting impression on me that surfaces daily. Whenever I am having a bad day, I think about Meaghan and somehow it's not so bad anymore. Meaghan was the most amazing person I have ever met.

Erin Duzan-Hachey (Meaghan's cousin)

Contents

Chapter 1 – A Life Changed Overnight… 5

Chapter 2 – The Diagnosis 17

Chapter 3 – Boston 31

Chapter 4 – The Trifecta: Chemo, Rehab, and Radiation 43

Chapter 5 – Be It Ever So Humble, There's No Place Like Home 55

Chapter 6 – The Good, The Bad And The Ugly 65

Chapter 7 – Here We Go Again 77

Chapter 8 – Collateral Damage 87

Chapter 9 – Death & Rebirth 97

Chapter 10 – Losing Ground… But Not Hope 123

Chapter 11 – Waiting for a Miracle 131

Chapter 12 – The Aftermath 149

Chapter 13 – Resuming Life 157

Chapter 14 – The Men in Meaghan's Life Speak 171

Chapter 15 – Meaghan Speaks 183

Chapter 16 – Life Lessons Learned 189

About The Author 191

Introduction: For Meaghan

Having a child with terminal cancer is a bi-polar expcrience because you constantly straddle two worlds, one of hope and one of reality. My beautiful daughter Meaghan was diagnosed with stage IV Glioblastomia Multiforme at the age of fourteen. Her type of cancer is usually found in the brain, but hers was rare and located in the central nervous system. Meaghan's journey was and is an inspiration to the scores of individuals who watched her blossom from a scared teenager into a courageous young woman. We made the journey together and had planned to write this book as a team, however the world of reality won out, and Meaghan became another pediatric cancer statistic. Meaghan always said that she did not want to be just "data" in a medical journal; she wanted to put a face with this disease. As Meaghan confronted her final days, she asked me to write this book alone to tell others how she lived, how she overcame challenges, how she excelled in the face of terminal illness, and ultimately who she was.

As I collect my thoughts, read my journals, and relive the days from initial diagnosis to her final breath, I realize that in many ways we were blessed. I was with Meaghan every day, and she was not alone in a hospital, as is unfortunately the case with many children. Although she had a brain tumor, it never affected her mind. Her personality, sense of humor and intelligence were always intact. Meaghan and I had a remarkable mother-daughter relationship that most would envy. We said "I love you" daily, and she thanked me constantly for helping her with the never-ending obstacles she encountered. She continued to smile her thousand-watt smile at everyone she met and never lost her long, thick, black hair (which was something she so dreaded). Meaghan was happy in spite of her medical condition. We laughed daily, embracing life without bitterness or anger. We were blessed with an abundance of help from friends, family members, and personal faith. Regardless of the twists and turns of her illness, Meaghan was never defeated. Every day, she worked toward her goal of beating the cancer and reclaiming the life that was stolen from her by this terrible disease.

Having cancer or having a child with cancer is cruel, unjust, and immediately life changing. Cancer is indiscriminate; it strikes without warning and touches all ages, genders, ethnicities, and economic backgrounds. Cancer knows no boundaries and bestows no mercy upon its victims. Having cancer or having a loved one with cancer is a life experience of tremendous personal growth. Having walked this journey alongside Meaghan, I will never again view the world the way I did prior to her diagnosis. I always knew that it was people, not material things, that are important in life, but walking this path made that lesson much clearer. As I reflect on photographs, letters, and memorabilia of Meaghan's life, each touches my heart and brings a smile to my face as I revisit each memory and return to the moment. Meaghan's life and death taught me to cherish each day and each memory for tomorrow is an uncertainty for all of us.

The summer before Meaghan was diagnosed with cancer, I was at Dana-Farber Cancer Institute with my sister, Karen, as she was in her second recurrence of stage IV breast cancer. We had gone to Boston for a second opinion with hope that they had a study or a more aggressive treatment than what she was currently receiving. The staff and physician were compassionate, competent, and professional, but ultimately they had no treatment to offer other than what she was receiving back home.

The doctor suggested that Karen have a brain scan, as her type of cancer has a tendency to spread. Although Karen had researched her type of breast cancer (Her2+), it had never occurred to her that the cancer could migrate to her brain. The very thought of it terrified her. We left Dana-Farber with mixed feelings; a world class cancer institution agreed with the treatment she was receiving at her local hospital, but her options were few, and the doctor was clear that the recurrence of her type of cancer was statistically not a good thing. After Karen's visit was completed, and as we were leaving the building, I looked at her and said, "This place sucks; it could only suck more if you were a child." Ironically, less than nine months later I would find myself back at Dana-Farber looking for an answer for my own child. The words continue to reverberate in my head, and I often wonder if I tempted fate or if it was God's way of showing me the path that we were to choose for Meaghan.

Once Meaghan was diagnosed with cancer, I spoke with my sister often. Their illnesses had eerily odd parallels; although I soon discovered that most aggressive cancers and their subsequent treatments have similarities. Meaghan and Karen were not unique, they were just experiencing the journey at the same time. In December of 2007, my sister lost her battle with cancer as it began to mutate against the chemotherapy and spread to different parts of her body, including what she feared most, her brain.

My husband, Jim, became an "expert of sorts" on glioblastomia. He researched the disease as soon as we learned it had a name. He learned early on that Meaghan's chances of beating this monster were not good. He educated himself on all current treatment options, ongoing research, and what drugs were in "study phases." Jim joined online groups to share and learn information on brain tumors and built an arsenal of research so if Meaghan had a recurrence, she would have options. When the first recurrence came, we did indeed have a "game plan," and Meaghan chose to fight as hard as she did a year earlier.

Meaghan's Story

Meaghan was able to participate in all decisions regarding her new treatment. We chose not to go back to Boston but went to Duke University Hospital in Durham, NC. (My sister was receiving treatment there as well.) Duke had an angiogenesis drug called Avastin, used in combination with a traditional chemotherapy Ironitecan (CPT 11), that showed great promise in beating glioblastomia's.

The drug worked for a short time, but one of the side effects of Avastin is blood clots, which Meaghan developed. The drug became too dangerous for her to continue. We were advised that stopping Avastin and continuing with Ironitecan alone might not contain the cancer. The doctors agreed that Meaghan needed to wait a minimum of three months before resuming the drug. We held our breath and prayed that Ironitecan would keep the cancer at bay. Jim continued his research, but the options, as in my sister's case, were experimental, and the risks to Meaghan's present and future health were in question. Regrettably, as was the case with my sister, Meaghan's cancer did recur and did so with a vengeance. When Meaghan was told the news that the cancer had spread, she handled the news with grace and told us that she wanted to live and asked that we find her a new treatment. She knew that her options were limited and completely understood the risks associated with an experimental drug, but she wanted to continue, whatever the consequence.

In the interim, we resumed life as we had come to know it. Once more we straddled the bi-polar world of terminal illness while we waited for either a miracle or the end. We never gave up hope and continued to look for a cure until her last day on this Earth.

Meaghan lost her battle to cancer on April 10, 2008, almost two years to the day after her initial diagnosis. However, her life, her spirit, her sense of purpose, her poetry, and her remarkable courage illustrate that she had won the war. I closed her eulogy with the following words:

"We are here to make ripples. Meaghan made waves."

Meaghan's was a life that was too short, but she made each minute count. I am honored to be her mother and honored to write her story.

Chapter 1 – A Life Changed Overnight...

> *On the average, 36 children and adolescents are diagnosed with cancer every day in the United States.*

March 2006 was going just how I had always thought life should be for people who are good parents, attend church, give to charity, and don't cheat on their taxes. I had returned to work after a twenty-year hiatus, and my husband Jim had switched jobs and was very content professionally as a traveling consultant. Our oldest son, Jimmy, was a sophomore at a local community college, working part-time, and planning to move away to a university in the fall. Our other two children were in high school. TJ was a junior and Meaghan a freshman, all three were doing well academically and socially and were happy, well-rounded teenagers. We had just purchased a new home and we were living the "American Dream," yet something kept nagging at me and waking me up at night. Something was amiss. I recall nightmares where I was burying a child; I never knew which child it was as the child was always faceless. I would wake up terrified and often in tears. I ignored the dreams and assumed they were just neurosis, because for once life seemed easy and pushed them to the back of my mind.

Meaghan, too, was having strange dreams about the death of one of her brothers. It varied from night to night, and being the irreverent individual I am, I told her it was just wishful thinking. She was also experiencing strange aches in her neck, knees, and shoulders and had an ominous feeling that something was terribly wrong with her. In her first fourteen years of life, Meaghan had always been very healthy and her only real medical problem was an occasional asthma attack. She had grown five inches in less than a year, so we assumed if anything, her pain was just adolescent growing pains and disregarded her fears as "teenage girl drama."

Near the end of March, Meaghan's high school, Grafton High, held its annual indoor field hockey tournament as a fundraiser for the senior prom. Since Meaghan played JV field hockey, she immediately signed up to play in the tournament. The fundraiser was open to all students, and a large number of freshmen decided to play, causing the JV

Janice Herrity

team to be split into two teams, leaving one team, her team, without a trained goalie. The coach decided that the fairest way to determine who would play goalie for each game would be to draw names from a hat. As luck would have it, Meaghan's name was drawn for one of the games.

    Meaghan hated playing goalie, but without objection she suited up and played the game. Once the game was finished, she burst into tears and ran from the court. I assumed her tears were from feeling solely responsible for the team's loss, so I went to find her and explain that all the girls had played poorly, not just her. I found her sitting in the locker-room sobbing and complaining not only of neck pain, but of pain throughout every inch of her body. I once more dismissed her pain as teenage drama and consoled her by telling her that once her last game was finished, we would go shopping - because retail therapy always heals a broken heart.

    The following week, Meaghan began having strange tingling sensations in both of her legs and a throbbing pain in her lower back. Track season was beginning, and she was having difficulty running four miles without her legs hurting. Meaghan came to me with her concerns and told me that she was thinking of quitting track because she was in so much pain. My response to her was that if she had not laid on the sofa all winter eating cupcakes, then perhaps she would be in better shape. Quitting might be something she would regret later, but ultimately it was her decision. The next day, Meaghan chose not to attend tryouts and came straight home, because she said that her pain was so intense that she knew she couldn't handle another demanding physical workout.

    Once home, Meaghan decided to rest, hoping that lying down would ease her pain. It did little to alleviate her suffering, so she decided to take a hot bath. Once she finished soaking, she tried to stand to get out of the tub, but her legs would not respond. After countless failed attempts, Meaghan eventually used her upper body strength and pulled herself over the side of the tub, cutting her leg open on the vanity nearby. Completely terrified, she wrapped herself in a towel, crawled to her bedroom, and immediately called me. Meaghan told me the events that had just transpired and although she sounded frightened, I again dismissed her fears and thought that this was just "Meaghan Drama." In fact, Meaghan drama happened so frequently that my cell phone ringer from home was a siren. I would answer the calls with the following greeting, "Drama phone, may I help you? What is your drama today?"

    I was stuck in traffic and since Meaghan was so adamant that she needed to see a doctor, I asked her to call my friend, Julia, and see if she could take Meaghan to the ER. I told Meaghan that she would need to wait in the parking lot for me to arrive because she was a minor and would need parental consent to be seen.

Meaghan's Story

I arrived about an hour later and found both Meaghan and Julia standing outside of Julia's van, laughing and eating take-out burgers. Meaghan showed absolutely no signs of anything seriously wrong, and I was very irritated that I had involved my friend in "Meaghan Drama." I admit I thought that Meaghan's complaints of physical pain were greatly exaggerated and that she was trying to avoid a problem at school with a "medical crisis." But since we were at the ER, seeing a doctor would be a good idea and hopefully would end her whining… however, I was not at all pleased about the hundred dollar co-pay.

Meaghan listed her symptoms for the doctor and told him that the pain had intensified since the field hockey tournament the weekend before. The ER doctor examined Meaghan and said that he could find nothing abnormal and thought she probably had pinched a nerve. He also said that the pressure from the hockey mask had most likely aggravated the problem. He saw no reason to order an X-ray or an MRI, so he prescribed pain killers and instructed us to call our primary care physician if the pain continued.

We filled the prescriptions and went home. I thought seeing a physician would calm Meaghan's fears, but it did not. She was still adamant that something was terribly wrong with her and asked me to feel the bump on the back of her neck. There was a large protrusion in the middle of her neck, and I had to admit that it was very odd. I tried to massage the area, but Meaghan said it hurt too much and asked me to stop. She again told me that she felt something was very wrong with her body, and once again I dismissed her fears. I presumed that the bump was most likely a knot caused by the tightness of the hockey mask and gave her a pain pill.

The following morning, Meaghan told me that her body really hurt, and she asked if she could stay home from school. I still thought her pain was more emotional than physical, so I agreed to a "mental health day." She looked at me and screamed, "I'm not faking! I really hurt, and I'm gonna call Dad. He'll believe me!" Then she promptly stomped to her room and slammed the door. Jim was working in Texas, and with the time difference, she awoke him at four-thirty in the morning. Meaghan asked him to take her to a real doctor because she hurt so badly and told him that I didn't believe her. After the initial shock of being awakened for another mother-daughter argument, Jim agreed to take her to another doctor if her pain continued. He told her that pinched nerves can be very painful and to stay home from school, get some rest, take her pain medication, and that he would be home later that evening. She then informed him that the medication did not help her pain and that the ER doctor was a "quack" and promptly slammed the phone down.

Janice Herrity

Meaghan slept most of that day and showed no signs that there was anything physically abnormal; but once again she said that she had a strange feeling that evening that something was terribly wrong with her. She came to me numerous times with her fears. Each time I told her it was a pinched nerve and that the pain would lessen in a few days. I also told her that if it continued, we would go see our primary care doctor for a second opinion.

Jim arrived home around one a.m. and found Meaghan awake in her room, kissed her goodnight, and told her not to let her fear get the best of her. The next morning she awoke around five. Since it was almost time for school, she decided to shake off her fears, shower, and begin her day. She got up, gathered her clean clothes, and while walking the short distance to the bathroom, collapsed. Her legs gave out on her, and she was once again unable to pull herself into a standing position. Absolutely terrified, she screamed for help. Her screams woke both Jim and me. We rushed to her aid, only to find her able to pull herself up and walk. We told Meaghan to take a pain pill, rest a little, and then shower. She then loudly reminded us that the pain pills didn't work, she wasn't faking, and that she had really fallen in the hallway. We looked at her, rolled our eyes, told her to "end the drama," and returned to bed.

A few minutes later, Meaghan tried once more to begin her day and fell a second time while getting out of bed. This time, TJ was awakened by her screams, and he and Jim helped Meaghan back into bed. It was April 14th (Good Friday), and there was a half day of school before Easter Break, so I told Meaghan to stay home and forget school. Since we all were awake, we began our day. I was showering and getting ready for work when Meaghan got up for a third and final time. Once again, she fell in the hallway. This time her screams were so loud that she woke Jimmy at the other end of the house. He ran to her aid and saw her lying in the hallway and asked Jim and TJ what was going on and why they were ignoring her. They explained that Meaghan had a pinched nerve so he should expect a fair amount of drama. In fact years before we had nicknamed Meaghan "Sarah Heartburn" because she was so dramatic, and we had had collectively learned to ignore her "crises." Jimmy looked at her and said, "Meaghan, if you were a horse, we'd shoot you," and went back to bed.

Meaghan continued to scream for help. She was inconsolable and demanding that we call an ambulance. Unlike the two previous falls, this time her legs would not respond, and she was unable to pull herself to her feet. We had no idea why Meaghan couldn't stand and assumed that she had broken a leg or hurt her back in the fall. We felt that if we moved her we could seriously injure her, so after much deliberation (all while Meaghan was screaming) we decided to call 911. Within minutes, the

Meaghan's Story

EMT's arrived. They did a quick assessment and could find no physical reason as to why Meaghan couldn't stand. They concluded that her pain and inability to bear weight was most likely due to a pinched nerve or a back injury. Her vital signs were normal, and there was no indication that there was anything seriously wrong with her, but the EMT's felt that Meaghan needed to be transported to the ER because she was in so much pain.

Jim followed the ambulance, and I finished showering. The oddest thing happened that morning while the EMT's were in the house: our dogs, who are not normally well behaved, sat quietly in a doorway while the EMT's attended to Meaghan. In fact, they were so quiet that we had forgotten that they were inside until they began to chase the ambulance as it pulled away. I often wonder if they could sense something we "more evolved species" could not.

I finished getting dressed, pushed my clients back an hour, and went to the hospital to assess the situation. The doctors and nurses assured me that Meaghan was fine and told me to leave, as she most likely had a pinched nerve, the same diagnosis we had received two days earlier.

As I got on the exit to go to Virginia Beach, an exit I had taken numerous times, somehow I got on the wrong entrance and headed west towards Williamsburg. I corrected my mistake and turned the car around and, oddly, ended up near the hospital. I went back to go east again only to repeat the same mistake, again ending up near the hospital. There was this voice inside telling me to cancel my appointment and stay, but I ignored it and finally got on the right exit and headed east, something I would later regret.

The first test that was ordered was an X-Ray of Meaghan's back. Since Meaghan was unable to move on her own, Jim held and positioned her so the technician could get the pictures he needed. The X-Ray showed everything was normal. The doctors still thought that Meaghan had a pinched nerve, but as a precaution, he ordered an MRI to ensure that there was not a neurological reason for her symptoms. I continued to call Jim to check on Meaghan, and he was getting very concerned because her pain was intensifying, and she was showing no signs of improvement. He suggested that I return to the hospital because Meaghan wasn't getting any better, and he was becoming very alarmed that something terrible might be happening with her.

I told my clients that I had to leave, and the moment I got on the interstate I ran into traffic. It was Good Friday, and the highways were totally gridlocked. I was not even half way to Yorktown (normally a forty-five minute drive) when my cell rang. It was Jim, he asked where I was, and I told him that I was stuck in traffic about four miles from the

Janice Herrity

Hampton Roads Bridge-Tunnel. The MRI results had come back. "It's bad," he said, "there's a tumor inside Meaghan's spinal cord."

I was stunned and in complete disbelief. How could she have a tumor? She had showed no signs of illness until a few days ago and had already been to an ER for a checkup. I then did what I always do when dealing with stress: I threw up. As luck would have it, I was strapped into my seat belt so I vomited all over myself. I continued to do so repeatedly for the next hour while driving in bumper-to-bumper traffic.

Jim told me that the doctors decided that Meaghan needed to be admitted to Children's Hospital of the Kings Daughters in Norfolk (CHKD), and a triage team was in transit to get her. He told me to go home, clean up, and then come to the ER. He said that the transport team had agreed to wait for me so I could accompany Meaghan and that he would drive separately and meet us at CHKD. Once I got home, I ran into the house, completely frantic, and informed the boys what was going on with their sister. I then told them that one of them would need to drive me to the hospital, and the other would need to clean my car as soon as possible. The boys took one look at me, covered with vomit, and began to argue who would be the "lucky one" to clean my car and who would drive me to the hospital.

I showered, grabbed the first thing I saw, and then called Jim and Meaghan to let them know that I would be there shortly. Jim said Meaghan was "holding her own" and that the triage team had not yet arrived, so there was no need to rush. Jimmy volunteered to drive me to the hospital. As he drove, I can still remember lecturing him on how nasty the inside of his car was and that I needed to throw up but the conditions and horrific smell prevented me from doing it.

I then went on a tirade on how he shouldn't smoke and the importance of a clean car, especially in case of emergencies... like if he needed to drive someone to a hospital! Afterward, I wondered why I was so concerned with the condition of his car while I had a child in crisis elsewhere. I suppose it's a normal mom reaction, or at least I hope it is.

Once I arrived at the ER, Jim told me that the triage team would be there any minute. They had been stuck in the same gridlock I had been in for the last two hours. I immediately went to see Meaghan, and the first words out of her mouth were, "Mom, are you okay?" I fell apart and started to cry, something that in the next few weeks would become commonplace for me when I wasn't vomiting. I was never a crier. I felt showing emotion in a crisis was both dramatic and a sign of weakness... however vomiting seemed oddly okay. I soon learned that tears are a sign of love and a reaction to deep pain. They would replace words in my life.

Meaghan's Story

The triage team arrived a few minutes later and began preparations to transport Meaghan to Norfolk. While they attended to Meaghan, Jim ushered Jimmy and me outside the examining room and began to educate us on her situation. He told us that the tumor appeared to be inside Meaghan's spinal cord and that the ER doctor had been in constant communication with CHKD. Meaghan would be taken directly to ICU for observation. The doctors felt she was too unstable for a floor and that there was a chance that they might operate later that evening. He told me that once we got to CHKD, the neurosurgeons would review the MRI and would talk with us afterward. He told Jimmy to go home and let TJ know what was happening and for both of them to stay home and wait for us to call.

We stood there shocked, sickened, and totally speechless. Then we all returned to Meaghan to assure her that everything was going to be fine. I had a hard time grasping the concept that this girl who had just run four miles earlier in the week now had a potentially life threatening tumor in her spine. As I write this passage over three years later, it is still inconceivable to me even that this scenario occurred.

The transport team assessed Meaghan's condition and then loaded her into the largest ambulance I had ever seen. There was an abundance of both medical equipment and supplies to ensure that the triage team would be prepared for any emergency that might occur while in transit. Meaghan was given Ativan at the ER and had fallen asleep, which was a good thing because once we left the hospital, we immediately became stuck in traffic amid all the vacationers heading east to Virginia Beach for Easter Break.

The interstate was completely gridlocked, so the ambulance driver tried an alternate route. It, too, was at a standstill, and it took us over an hour to go just ten miles. I asked the driver why he was only using the ambulance's flashing lights and not the sirens to get us out of this mess. To my surprise, he replied that sirens cause people to panic and that driving with both sirens and lights is more dangerous than lights alone. Plus, he needed authorization to use both.

This was my first real foray into the medical world, and I would soon learn that most of my preconceived notions of hospitals, doctors, nurses, therapists, and insurance companies were wrong. Meaghan woke up while in transport to CHKD and asked where she was and if I was with her. The nurses told her I was in the front seat, and she was on her way to Kings Daughters. I spoke to her, and she smiled and fell back to sleep. I then called my mother to inform her of Meaghan's condition, only to find out later that I was so emotional that she had no idea what I was saying.

Janice Herrity

Once we arrived at CHKD, Meaghan was rushed to ICU. Within minutes of her arrival, she was connected to all types of machines to monitor her medical condition. Each was foreign to me, but within a few months, I would be able to identify each machine, tell you its purpose, understand the data, and even calibrate dosages in milligrams.

Jim arrived while I was filling out paperwork, and he met with the neurosurgeon. The neurosurgeon told him that the plan was to begin the steroid Decadron immediately to reduce the swelling in Meaghan's spinal cord and that an MRI had been ordered for the next day to get a clearer picture of what was happening with her central nervous system.

ICU was nothing like what is depicted on television. Meaghan, along with perhaps twenty-five other children, was in a ward of sorts, separated only by curtains. Each nurse was responsible for two patients. The nurses sat at a desk between the two patients' cubicles, monitored the machines, and were only steps away from the patients in case an emergency should arise.

The only word to describe ICU is "chaotic" - machines beeping, a whirlwind of medical personnel, and dazed parents trying to grasp the shock of a seriously ill child. There are no windows, only bright florescent lights, and you never know what time of day it is. In a way, the atmosphere is very similar to a casino, but the gambling is life or death.

When I reflect upon that first night. I can only compare it to being in a foxhole during war. You're perhaps closer to God than ever before, praying constantly for your child's survival, and the intense fear that you experience is so powerful and palpable that it changes you as a person. We met one family whose child had been in ICU for over a month, the little boy was four and had cancer. The family had a great deal of support. His mother told me that what got her through the endless tough days were the Three F's: Friends, Family and Faith. I never forgot her words, and we would also experience that the Three F's were the key to surviving our nightmare.

By midnight, Jim and I were exhausted, both physically and emotionally. The hospital policy was that both parents could be in ICU with their child, but they must be awake at all times. If you needed to sleep, there were beds in the ICU parents' lounge. Jim urged me go to sleep, and since Meaghan was asleep and holding her own, I agreed to go with the one stipulation that we would switch around three o'clock in the morning.

When I returned for my shift, Meaghan was wide-awake asking why "Papa" was in the corner of her room (Papa was Jim's father and had passed away three years earlier). Meaghan said that he was wearing his lime green shorts, white polo shirt, baseball cap, and sneakers (Strangely

Meaghan's Story

the afterlife hadn't upgraded his wardrobe). She told us that he had not spoken to her but continued to stand nearby, just watching. Jim and I just looked at each other, astonished and somewhat frightened, not afraid of Jim's dad, but at the very idea that only Meaghan could see him. At first we dismissed her vision as a reaction to the drugs, but as the evening progressed, both Jim and I became believers that indeed his deceased father was present. I even told Jim to tell his Dad to leave and that Meaghan wasn't going anywhere with him tonight or anytime soon. I then threw a pillow at the empty corner, which in retrospect is rather amusing, because if Jim's dad could travel through the time and space continuum, surely a hospital pillow wouldn't have harmed him.

The next day we waited patiently for a call for Meaghan's MRI and were very anxious to see if the steroids had begun to reduce the swelling in her spinal cord. Around one in the afternoon, radiology phoned Meaghan's nurse and said that there was an opening in the schedule and that they were ready for Meaghan. In order to transport Meaghan to radiology, the nurses had to pack up everything in her cubicle and make each machine portable. The procedure took close to ten minutes, and as the nurse was pushing Meaghan out of ICU, the phone rang a second time and her nurse was informed that she had taken too long to get Meaghan downstairs, so her slot was given to another patient. The nurse then unpacked everything, plugged the machines back in, and waited patiently for another open slot.

I still remember my disbelief that a patient in ICU was just another patient on the log, and I learned Lesson I: Time is money, and a hospital (even a children's hospital) is a business. This revelation would be useful as I learned to advocate for our daughter, and it served me well.

A few hours later, ICU received another call from radiology that they were once again ready for Meaghan. Her nurse once more began packing up Meaghan's cubicle. While in the process of making all the machines portable, radiology called a second time and informed her nurse that if she was not there in five minutes, the technicians would move on to another patient. Frustrated, the nurse went to radiology to guarantee Meaghan's spot was saved. Meanwhile, the other ICU nurses finished packing her machines.

I remember asking the nurses why Meaghan needed all this medical equipment. They told me that they needed to be prepared. In the event that an emergency occurred outside of ICU, they would be able to respond rapidly. After the MRI was completed, we met with one of the neurosurgeons, and he confirmed the results of the previous MRI.

He informed us that the tumor was approximately six centimeters (two and a half inches) and was located in the cervical area of Meaghan's spinal cord. He said that there was a great deal of swelling in the cord, so he would need to operate as soon as possible. He was hoping for Monday morning, but he had not ruled out the possibility that they may need to operate sooner.

When we returned to ICU, two priests from our parish and Meaghan's youth minister were waiting to perform the Sacrament of Healing for the Sick/Last Rites. Priests are to refrain from sacraments on Holy Saturday, but in Meaghan's case they made an exception because she was so very ill and because Meaghan wanted the sacrament. Before the priest began the sacrament, Meaghan told him, "That better not be Last Rites, because I'm not going anywhere." Meaghan was very comforted that they came, and their presence helped put her at ease.

We met with one of the neurosurgeons again on Sunday. He assured us that they had done this type of operation before and expected the surgery to take approximately six hours. However, he warned us that once the surgeons got "inside" and looked through the surgical binocular microscope, things could change. The surgeon explained that the procedure would involve cutting through Meaghan's flesh and tissue and then they would need to saw open her backbone to reach her spinal cord. After they reached the cord, they would operate with tweezers to remove the tumor, hoping to avoid as much damage to the spinal cord and central nervous system as possible. The neurosurgeon then went on to explain how messages travel through the spine, as if we were idiots. But we both just listened to the anatomy lesson.

As he was talking, I remember thinking, tweezers, they're going to operate with tweezers? I cannot even tweeze my eyebrows without screwing up, and how the hell are they going to do this! We agreed to the operation and, oddly, had few questions. We felt we had no choice and signed the consent forms.

It never occurred to either Jim or me to look into the option of having Meaghan moved to another hospital for the surgery. Even if we had, I am not sure she could have endured the trip. As a write this passage three years later, it is my greatest regret that we did not look into larger medical hospitals for her surgery. CHKD did a great job, and they saved Meaghan's life, but I just wish we had covered all our options. I often wonder why no other hospital was presented as an option for a surgery of this nature. There are larger medical centers like UVA, Johns Hopkins, and Duke within a few hours travel time. Duke, we learned later on in our journey, has an MRI in the operating room to assist the surgeon.

I often wonder if I would I be co-authoring this book with Meaghan if we had gone elsewhere. I also know that if we had gone somewhere else, we might have had overly zealous neurosurgeons and

Meaghan's Story

Meaghan could have been left a paraplegic. I realize that you have to play the cards you are dealt, and we most likely would not have chosen another hospital. Nevertheless, I regret not looking into it and am angered that we were not offered the option.

Chapter 2 – The Diagnosis

> *On the average, one in every four elementary schools has a child with cancer. The average high school has two students who are current or former cancer patients.*

Early Monday morning, the surgical team arrived in ICU and began preparations for the operation. Over the weekend Meaghan's condition had stabilized, and the MRI results indicated that the steroids had reduced some of the swelling in the spinal cord. Jim and I met briefly with the neurosurgeons, and they reviewed the surgical procedure one last time. Both were confident that Meaghan would handle the surgery with relative ease because she was in such good physical condition, but they warned that surgical complications could never be ruled out. We had very few questions and then returned to ICU just as the team was beginning to move Meaghan to the operating room. I asked her if she was frightened and she said, "No. I just want to get this thing out of me, and with any luck I'll be back at school in time for state testing."

We followed the gurney to an area of the corridor that was posted "staff only," kissed her forehead, and told her that we loved her. As the nurses were wheeling Meaghan into the operating room, we heard her ask the one of the surgeons if he had marked the area he intended to operate on, because she had read about surgical errors where surgeons had operated on the wrong body part. He replied that he had it "under control." Meaghan then asked if he had ever been sued for malpractice.

Once Meaghan was out of sight, I sat down in the hallway and wept. Jim and I were directed to the surgical waiting room where we were told that a nurse would call us every hour to let us know how the surgery was progressing and how Meaghan was holding up. It was a little before eight in the morning when we entered the waiting room. It was full of anxious parents nervously awaiting the results of their child's surgery.

Janice Herrity

Time moves slowly when you are waiting for an answer to a pressing issue. Imagine waiting to hear the results of a major surgery on your child – time moves at a snail's pace. At first I tried to fill the time with reading a book, but I was unable to focus and never got past the first page. Since reading didn't distract me, I quickly moved on to eating. I went downstairs to the cafeteria where I ran into one of the neurosurgeons who happened to be in line in front of me. I was completely stunned to see him, so I asked why he wasn't in the operating room. He explained that due to the length of the operation, the surgeons were taking turns and that he would take over once the other surgeon got Meaghan open. Then he ordered his breakfast of biscuits with sausage gravy. I remember thinking to myself he's a doctor; doesn't he know that crap will kill him? Then being the health nut that I am, I ordered my breakfast of scrambled eggs with cheddar cheese, bacon, sausage, biscuits and two sides of corn beef hash.

After finishing my breakfast, I returned to the waiting area and turned my attention to vending machine food, terrible hospital coffee, and stale Girl Scout cookies. Jim filled his time somewhat more productively by researching spinal cord tumors and telecommuting to his job in Texas.

Most of the other children's surgeries took an hour or so. The surgeon would appear in the waiting room and tell the worried parent that the operation had gone beautifully and that they could soon see their child in the recovery room. We overheard many of the conversations. Most of the children were having minor operations like having tubes inserted or removed in their ears. By noon, only Jim and I, along with a hospital volunteer, remained in the waiting room. Just a few hours earlier this same room had been bustling with activity, but now it was completely silent except for the occasional ring of the telephone. Each time the phone rang, the hospital volunteer called our name. Each call was exactly the same, the operating room nurse would calmly tell us the same scripted bull that they tell everyone – that Meaghan's surgery was progressing nicely and she was holding her own.

Around three-thirty, one of the neurosurgeons appeared in the waiting area and told us they were done and that the other surgeon was "closing her up" and that Meaghan would soon be moved to recovery. We were told that we would be able to see her within the hour. He then said that he had no idea what type of tumor was in her spine but that it had been sent to pathology for analysis. Most importantly, he thought he had removed it all. Relieved and elated, we thanked the surgeon and waited for the call to go to the recovery room. As promised, within the hour we were told we could go see Meaghan. Once we entered the recovery room, we were told that Meaghan was conscious and had just punched

Meaghan's Story

the other neurosurgeon upon waking. The doctor was laughing and said, "Most of my patients wake up and thank me" but he welcomed the slug. It meant that she was a "Fighter."

Once it was determined that Meaghan was not going to have any surgical complications, she returned to ICU. The following days were absolutely horrific. Jim and I were completely unprepared for the amount of pain that Meaghan was in. We were unable to help her, other than to voice our despair over the entire situation.

Meaghan was unable to move her head even inches without screaming in pain, and the morphine did little to ease her suffering. She was unable to sit up or move her legs, and she was rapidly losing muscle mass. Each day we saw a horde of doctors, including surgeons, neurologists, physiatrists (a fancy name for a rehab doctor), residents, and interns. With each examination, we asked the doctors what type of tumor was removed and if they knew if it was malignant or benign. They all told us the same thing – that the tumor had been sent to Mayo Clinic for neuropathology and that they should have an answer in a day or two. Both Jim and I were certain that the doctors had preliminary data, and we became extremely irritated that they did not share the information with us. Each doctor that examined Meaghan pricked her toes to see if she had feeling. She did, and she was even able to wiggle a few. The physicians were encouraged that she was able to respond to the sensation of touch, and her ability to move her toes indicated that her nervous system was intact and processing messages.

Within days of the surgery, Meaghan began to show signs of stabilization and improvement, but she was still unable to move her legs, she had lost the ability to hold her feet upward, and her legs were beginning to turn to the side. Unaware that there was an orthopedic device to correct the problem, I found my own solution by propping pillows, blankets, and towels around her ankles to hold her feet up. I was so concerned about her feet that I pointed it out to each doctor that examined her. I suspect that they were so sick of hearing me complain that they sent a physical therapist to fit Meaghan for special boots.

The boots were made of sheepskin and had kickstands on the back that kept Meaghan's legs straight and kept her feet from flopping to the side. Once I got Meaghan's feet and legs under control, I turned my attention to nagging the doctors about her rapid loss of muscle mass and about when she could eat solid food again because she was extremely hungry. Because Meaghan was immobile, she needed to be connected to a machine that contracted her leg muscles and pushed the blood back to her heart to prevent blood clots. She was also attached to a number of other machines that monitored her oxygen level, heart rate, blood pressure, and bodily fluids, as well as IV fluids, IV medications, and a morphine pump.

My heart broke for her. There was nothing Jim or I could do to help her or alleviate her suffering, and there was an intense sadness in her eyes. Meaghan was helpless, and we were powerless. I made a vow to myself that day that I would never let her dignity be compromised. I kept that vow until the day she died.

The doctors ordered another MRI to view Meaghan's spine post-surgery. To avoid the same problem that we had with the previous MRI, we asked one of the ICU doctors to call radiology and explain Meaghan's situation and request patience while the nurses prepared Meaghan for transport.

Unlike the previous MRI, this time we accompanied Meaghan to radiology and once there were instructed to go to a waiting area adjacent to the MRI room. We did as requested, but that would be the last time we would ever leave Meaghan's side. We could hear the nurses and technicians in the next room, and suddenly we heard Meaghan scream. Jim jumped up and ran to the next room and found Meaghan in tears. He asked what happened, and the technician replied that in order to get the proper angle, he had to grab Meaghan's neck. Meaghan then told Jim that pain shot through every inch of her body when the technician grabbed her neck. Jim "politely" told the technician to be extremely gentle as she had just had major surgery. He understood the need to get the pictures, but if he hurt her again he was going to inflict similar pain on him; I still am amazed that the hospital personnel did not call security on him! That day we learned Lesson II: As a parent, you have rights and can accompany your child or loved one anywhere in a hospital, with the exception of the operating room.

Jim and I had been in the hospital world for over a week and the "deer in the headlights response" had worn off. We knew we had rights, so that evening we demanded to see the MRI pictures. The resident on duty pulled up the scans on a computer in the ICU, and what we saw shocked us. The scan clearly showed two white images on the screen. We knew at once that the white images meant that there were still two tumors in Meaghan's spinal cord.

We were both absolutely flabbergasted. Up until that moment, we were under the impression that the surgeons had removed the entire tumor. The two tumors that remained were undetected on the earlier MRI's due to the amount of swelling in Meaghan's spinal cord. The resident on duty then explained that the tumor had metastasized, which we knew was the worst-case scenario. Lesson III: Do not assume that a resident will be able to give you accurate information just because he or she is a doctor. Wait for someone who has finished their training to inform you of tests results.

We knew we needed to tell Meaghan the results before she heard it from the hospital personnel, so later that evening we broke the news to Meaghan. She was brokenhearted and inconsolable and told us that her pain was so intense that she did not think she could endure another surgery.

The doctors finally changed Meaghan's orders to allow her to eat solid food. She asked Jim to go to Wendy's and get her a cheeseburger, fries, and shake. While Jim was gone, one of the surgeons came to check on Meaghan and I asked him again if the results of the pathology report were back. He said, "Yes."

I asked if it was cancer and he replied, "Yes, and it's a very aggressive form." He went on to tell me that her type of cancer was very rare in the spine and her "chance of survival was very poor, perhaps six months." Fortunately, Meaghan was out of earshot and did not hear our conversation. I fell to the floor sobbing and ran out of the ICU so she would not see me crying.

I immediately called Jim, who was in line at Wendy's, to inform him of the test results. I still have no idea why I didn't wait until he returned to update him. I suppose it was a knee-jerk reaction from shock. Jim arrived a few minutes later with Meaghan's lunch. I was completely amazed that he was able to contain his emotions and get her food. He said regardless of the pathology results, Meaghan was hungry, he promised her a burger, and he was going to fulfill her wish.

Before reentering the ICU, we quickly discussed when would be the appropriate time to tell Meaghan the horrendous news. We felt that she needed to hear the test results from us before someone from the hospital told her. We asked the physicians to not discuss her pathology results with her until we talked with her privately.

That evening, Jim and I told Meaghan that she had cancer. She looked at us and replied in a matter of fact tone, "Yeah, I thought so. I saw mom having a meltdown earlier." We told her that we were going to have a meeting with the oncologist once he returned from vacation, so we would learn more then. We also asked her if she wanted to be present. She replied, "Yes." The news was devastating, but Meaghan handled it better than we did.

Ten days after being admitted to the ICU, Meaghan was well enough to be moved to a step-down unit. This unit of the hospital is designed for patients who no longer required the intense nursing of ICU but are still not strong enough for a regular floor.

Janice Herrity

Since Meaghan wanted to be included in the meeting, the oncologist agreed to meet with us in the step-down unit. My sister, Karen, and her husband came up from North Carolina to see Meaghan and joined in the meeting. Karen had been battling stage IV breast cancer for almost two years, and we felt that her assistance and knowledge would be invaluable. She lived in this world, and she understood the language, and more importantly, the emotions we were all feeling. We felt that we needed her experience and input to help us navigate our situation.

Once Meaghan was settled, we met with the oncologist that specialized in brain and spinal cord tumors to go over a treatment plan. To help ease the tension in the room, the oncologist made a stupid joke. It backfired, and Meaghan began to cry… then the meeting began. We all learned later that his dim-witted humor was part of his personality. Meaghan grew to love him along with his bad jokes, and more importantly she trusted him with her life. He explained that Meaghan's type of tumor was a Glioblastomia Multiforme (GBM), a brain tumor that had developed in her central nervous system. It was grade IV and extremely rare in the spine. The two tumors that remained were not metastasis, but tentacles. He explained that this type of tumor spreads by tentacles and is very aggressive. He told us that although two tumors remained, the surgeons advised against another surgery.

The oncologist explained that with this type of tumor, we needed to start chemotherapy and radiation as soon as possible and then afterward address the paralysis. Once Meaghan was strong enough, she would be released from the hospital, and chemotherapy and radiation would be done on an outpatient basis.

We all were overwhelmed by her diagnosis. I remember asking the doctor where Meaghan would get radiation. The oncologist replied in a matter-of-fact tone, "Norfolk General," which is adjacent to CHKD. I explained that this plan seemed completely impractical, as it had taken us two and a half hours to get to CHKD in an ambulance and Meaghan was unable to sit up and was in tremendous pain.

I left the meeting and sat outside ICU and cried hysterically. My heart actually ached, and my chest heaved with each breath. I feel like my heart literally broke. It was such a deep pain and so incredibly intense that there were no words to describe it. Through my tears, I kept repeating the same words to my sister, "How am I going to do this? How am I going to be able to help Meaghan? How am I going to get her there each day? She cannot even sit up." That was the first time that I realized that the bulk of Meaghan's medical care and recovery would become my responsibility. I had no training. What would happen to Meaghan if I failed?

Meaghan's Story

As I sat in that hallway and sobbed, I had an epiphany of sorts. I knew in my heart that Meaghan needed to go to a hospital that would give her chemotherapy, radiation, and rehabilitation all at the same time and that we needed to leave home to get it. Meaghan was an athlete with an athlete's mind, and the sooner we attacked the problem, the sooner she would heal physically, mentally, and emotionally.

I knew Meaghan well enough to know that although it was not the standard treatment to attack this monster all at once, that's what Meaghan would want and that's what she needed. I knew that fighting a serious illness is as much a mental battle as it is a physical one, so we needed to get her in the right mental state by attacking the paralysis and the cancer at the same time.

Jim had written down all the information that the oncologist had provided and he, too, came to the same conclusion – that Meaghan would need to be treated in a research hospital. He was sending informational emails to St. Jude's, M.D. Anderson, and Dana Farber to see if they could treat the cancer and get Meaghan rehabilitation at the same time. Meanwhile, my brother-in-law was on his computer researching glioblastomia. He confirmed that the survival rates were very poor, and the limited information on GBM in the spine was dismal.

Meaghan asked us to leave her alone. She said that she needed to call her best friend Katie and talk to her. I was on the other side of the curtain, and all I could hear was a sobbing brokenhearted teenage girl telling her best friend that she had cancer and might die. After Meaghan finished her phone call, she was absolutely hysterical, so the resident ordered Valium to calm her down and help her rest. The Valium caused an interaction with the morphine, and Meaghan began to struggle to breathe. Machines and monitors began beeping, and alarms began to sound. I can still recall the horror on Meaghan's face as she was simultaneously gasping for air and praying to God to end her nightmare and put her out of her misery.

The medical staff reacted quickly to counteract the drug interaction, and within a short time, Meaghan began to breathe normally once again. As parents, Jim and I had never felt as helpless and powerless as we did that moment. I can still remember Jim's words to me, "We have to find a way to not let this make us bitter, or we will never be able to help her."

It had been a little over ten days since this thing first reared its ugly head, and Meaghan's life had literally changed overnight… and the world we once knew no longer existed.

The following day, Meaghan was moved to the oncology floor. She had a spacious private room with a lovely view of the Lafayette River.

Janice Herrity

We watched the ships going up to the terminal each day. Life on the hospital floor was very peaceful compared to the madness of the ICU.

Meaghan could now have visitors, and one of us was able to stay with her in the room. There was a private bath, and life was less chaotic. I was adamant that Meaghan have a bath and get her hair washed, but the doctors said that she was too weak, so I gave her a sponge bath. Her hair was knotted and caked with dried blood from the surgery. I was told that she could not get the steri-strips on the back of her neck wet, so with the help of a nurse's aide, I washed her hair with a dry shampoo.

Meaghan was thrilled to be clean and looked forward to having visitors and seeing people other than hospital personnel. She asked Jim to go to the mall and get her some clothes. Meaghan had been in hospital gowns for eleven days, and she wanted some age appropriate clothing. I, too, had been in the same clothing for days and was sure those around me wanted me in clean clothes, so I asked Jim to pick me up a few things as well. He agreed to do our shopping and headed straight to Victoria's Secret for Meaghan and thankfully he found a sales associate to assist him. He returned with adorable sweat outfits, underwear, and pajamas, all in Meaghan's size.

Jim chose Kmart for my clothing needs and returned with two shirts from the maternity department, clearance underwear with smiley faces on the behind, socks from the children's department, and a hunter green sweatshirt embellished with both teddy bears and hearts, highlighted with huge lettering that read "Norfolk." I was in such need of clean clothes that, sadly, I wore some of the things that he purchased.

Meaghan's visitors came in droves and filled her room with uproarious laughter. Their visits helped her to forget her situation, and for a short time, she felt like a normal teenager. Jim and I had visitors as well, and we were overwhelmed by the outpouring of support and love from family and friends. Our sons came to see Meaghan for the first time and were absolutely shocked by their sister's condition, but within a few minutes they all exchanged insults with one another, and normalcy returned to their sibling relationship.

The boys asked me to tell people to stop bringing food. They said that neighbors and family friends had been bringing meals by the house for days and they didn't need anything else. Jimmy said that when he returned from school earlier that day, he had found four lasagnas in the fridge, and our neighbor's grandmother was vacuuming the family room. She had already run the dishwasher and was making them a pot roast!

I asked them what they ate for dinner as they had numerous choices and an abundance of food, and their reply was, "We ordered pizza." I could not believe it! A house full of food and they ordered out…

typical. Meaghan then loudly suggested that they consider locking the front door so the evil lasagna and pot roast people could not just walk in!

We saw fewer and fewer doctors now that Meaghan was on the oncology floor. That was not a bad thing, but the neurologist informed us during one of his examinations that the chances were slim that Meaghan would ever walk again. His words were, and I quote, "The spinal cord has limited ability to heal itself." Meaghan began to cry, and we were all overwhelmed by his words. I remember thinking, "Who gets cancer and loses the ability to walk overnight?" It made no sense!

Meaghan became furious with the doctor and wanted us to fire him from her case. Her rage was the first positive sign we had seen in her since the surgery. The fact that she was angry enough to fight made us very happy. It showed us that although her body was damaged, her personality was still intact.

After the neurologist left, Meaghan looked at me and said, "I know why this happened to me; it's because I lied during confession." I looked and her and said, "Meaghan, everybody lies during confession. This is not a punishment from God. There was a mistake in your DNA, and your RNA kept repeating the mistake. You did nothing to bring this on."

She looked at me and said, "You really think everyone lies to the priest?"

I said, "Maybe not everyone - maybe ninety-five percent, either by flat out lying or by a sin of omission; however I think the nuns are a pretty safe bet for telling the truth."

Meaghan laughed and said, "Yeah, I know it's random, but why me?"

I looked at her and said, "Why not you? No one is immune from the injustice of life. It just sucks that it's you and not me." I also told her that people beat cancer every day and that statistics are just numbers. Someone has to be the one to beat the odds, and her dad and I were betting on her. I also told her that doctors are wrong all the time and that they always give the patient the worst case scenario so that the patient will not have false hope and perhaps, more importantly, so they cannot be sued later on! I told her to ignore the neurologist's words, get in touch with her "Inner Diva," and show him he was mistaken. I also told her that he was not only a doctor but also a father and a human being, and he would be overjoyed if he were wrong.

The next morning we met a physical therapist named Christine. She told Meaghan to "never give up hope and with hard work and a positive attitude anything is possible." That day with help from both

Janice Herrity

Christine and the occupational therapist, Meaghan stood for the first time since she fell in our hallway two weeks earlier. Although she had assistance and stood for only seconds, the experience changed Meaghan's mental outlook, and she looked at me and said, "I am going to beat this thing, and I am going to walk again and reclaim my life."

The following day, Meaghan was able to sit in a wheelchair for the first time. Soon her body began to respond to cues, and she began to have limited feeling return to both her toes and legs. The physical therapists came daily and taught me how to help Meaghan exercise in bed so she could keep her muscle tone and retain both range and motion in her legs. Within a few days, Meaghan began to move parts of her body on her own with no assistance. Although two tumors remained, her spinal cord was responding to voluntary and involuntary messages, and her surgery was successful.

Jim and I found it very difficult to sit back and trust complete strangers with our daughter's life, so we continued to look into treatment options for her illness. We soon learned Lesson IV: Hospitals and insurance companies control just about everything regarding treatment, and they expect a fair amount of compliance from the patient and the families in return.

I still find it odd that so many people do not question the medical community and just assume that doctors will have the right solution for their loved one. In retrospect, they are the professionals, and most of them are proficient. They have the contacts and knowledge to work within the framework of each patient's diagnosis and individual insurance plan. However, with our child, we were going to ensure that we took the lead in the decision making process. Initially we thought that Meaghan would receive her treatment at St. Jude's, but our insurance company felt that Meaghan should go to Dana-Farber Cancer Institute in Boston. There was an open study, and the doctors had treated a spinal GBM before. The insurance company was pushing for treatment at Dana-Farber in Boston and was on their list as a "Center of Excellence." Lesson V: We were not in control.

Our next challenge was getting Meaghan into the study. Dana-Farber is part of the Harvard Medical system, which includes Massachusetts General Hospital, Brigham & Women's Hospital, Spaulding Rehabilitation, and Boston Children's Hospital. All are world renown, and it seemed like an excellent fit for Meaghan's situation. Jim's niece, Erin, is a nurse at Mass General, so she was able to contact the person in charge of the study and see if Meaghan fit the study parameters.

Both Jim and our oncologist at CHKD contacted Dana-Farber and were told that they would accept Meaghan as a patient. They agreed to include rehabilitation along with chemo and radiation. The oncology social worker at CHKD contacted a non-profit group called Air Compassion of America to transport Meaghan to Boston since she was physically unable to take a commercial flight.

Our next obstacle was high school. Meaghan was terrified that she would fall behind and not graduate with her class. I called Grafton High and spoke with the principal. She was aware that Meaghan was very ill and already had a plan in motion. The principal had contacted each of Meaghan's teachers to see where they were in their lesson plans and what was needed to meet the state requirements. State testing was scheduled in two weeks, and most classes were in review, so Meaghan was closed out for the year and became a sophomore.

However, there was one stipulation: once things settled down, Meaghan would need to take the Virginia state mandated tests because they were a requirement for graduation. Now that I had Meaghan's educational concerns taken care of, I turned my attention to our son, TJ. I explained to the principal that most likely Meaghan and I would be leaving within the next few days for Boston, and Jim was working in Texas, leaving TJ alone with Jimmy. This could be a potential disaster. She agreed to let TJ drive to school so he could have transportation for after school activities and sports. She also told me that she would talk with TJ's teachers and tell them to keep an eye on him. I was very concerned about leaving TJ, but we had no choice. We quickly learned Lesson VI: When someone in the family is diagnosed with cancer, they do not get it alone. The whole family gets cancer.

TJ was to be confirmed at our parish, and although I wanted to attend, I felt that I needed to stay with Meaghan. Adding to my dilemma, I was a mentor for another confirmation candidate and was required to be present for her. Fortunately, the young woman was a family friend and was aware of Meaghan's situation. She was able to find a substitute mentor to assume my role.

Jim decided that he would go and support TJ, so he went home for the first time in over two weeks to inspect the damage done to the house by the boys, freeze the abundance of food, do laundry, and get a good night's sleep.

We were all feeling rather optimistic about the future. In a matter of a few days we seemed to have found the right mix of hospitals, gotten school off the plate, and taken care of the boys. Then it hit me - in the midst of this craziness, we had to move! We had planned to rent our current house, but it became very clear that we needed to put our house up for sale because we needed the equity to pay the medical bills, and I wouldn't be around to pack or keep the house in order for showings.

Janice Herrity

Thankfully, my niece Jessica, volunteered to come and help out. She was in her junior year at Canisius College in Buffalo and would come to Virginia as soon as her exams were finished. Her gracious offer let me relax so I could focus all my attention on Meaghan.

Nevertheless, new problems arrived daily. The first of which was that Meaghan began to run a low-grade temperature and had a great deal of blood in her urine. She had developed a urinary tract infection (UTI). This would be the first of many UTI's that Meaghan would continually experience over the next two years. It is a common problem for people who have spinal cord injuries because the injury interferes with the nerve messages between the brain and the sphincter muscle. The muddled messages resulted in Meaghan's bladder's inability to completely empty, allowing bacteria to enter and multiply. Meaghan was paralyzed from the waist down, so she also had to retrain both her bladder and bowels. This was very difficult and humiliating for her, but she was determined not to live her life wearing a diaper. She set her mind to overcoming the obstacle and retrained both within a few months.

In addition to the urinary tract infection, the shock to Meaghan's system was wearing off, and she began to experience continual nerve pain. The morphine pump did little to help with Meaghan's neuropathic pain. She was prescribed a drug called Neurontin. The doctors were positive that the drug would work but warned that it could take days, maybe weeks, to get into Meaghan's system. In the interim, she would have to deal with the pain. Meaghan described the pain as "relentless and intense" and said that it ran up her legs, crossed her abdomen, and then shot back down to her toes. The intensity of neuropathic pain often came with spasms, which Meaghan experienced daily. One episode lasted for over eighteen hours. Jim and I discovered that massage helped with the neuropathy, so we took turns massaging Meaghan's legs and putting ice packs on her toes to relieve the burning sensation of the nerve pain.

Meaghan continued to do range of motion leg exercises even through the pain. As an athlete, she knew that she needed to use her muscles or they would deteriorate. She began to push through the pain to accomplish her goal of walking again. Meaghan worked so hard that two and a half weeks after surgery, she was able to sit alone on the edge of the bed for two and a half minutes, and she stood on the parallel bars with assistance for one minute. These new milestones gave us hope and got us through the toughest of days. The advice given to us early in the ICU was to "take life one day at a time." It turned out to be the best advice we ever received, but at times it seemed like we were taking life one hour or one minute at a time.

What got us through those first few weeks were Friends, Family and Faith. The Three F's were central to our survival. I often wondered

Meaghan's Story

how people who were alone and had little faith survived a crisis. Our friends came each day and brought us coffee and food from our favorite restaurants. We did not have to leave the hospital or eat cafeteria food. Our friends checked on the boys, cleaned the house, mowed the lawn, and tried to remove as many obstacles as they could from our lives.

Meaghan's friends were just as terrific – her hospital room was filled with flowers, balloons, stuffed animals, movies, books, t-shirts, and posters. We were never at a loss for visitors, and they continually lifted our spirits. Prior to us leaving for Boston, we sent home four carloads of gifts, as we could not take everything with us. My friend Kim was helping me pack up Meaghan's belonging as we were preparing to leave CHKD, and I came across a clump of Meaghan's hair that had been cut from her head for the surgery. We looked at each other, I sighed, and then I just threw it out. I regret that now. I wish I had kept it, so I could have a piece of her to hold.

Chapter 3 – Boston

> *Cancer is the leading cause of death by disease in children under the age of 15 in the United States.*

The following morning, Meaghan was discharged from CHKD. It had been a little over two weeks since this nightmare began, and Meaghan and I both had mixed emotions about leaving Norfolk to receive treatment in Boston. Meaghan was already missing her room, her dogs, her friends, and her brothers, and she was apprehensive about the loneliness that she would feel away from familiar surroundings. I, too, was hesitant, but I could not allow my mind to go to that place. I needed to be strong and reassure her that Boston was the right choice for her treatment. We had come to respect and trust the doctors and nurses at this hospital, but we needed to go where they had seen this type of cancer before. It was imperative that we go to a hospital with the latest research and clinical studies in order to save her life.

We left CHKD around eight-thirty in the morning. Due to the weight restrictions aboard the plane, we were each allowed only one bag, which could not exceed fifty pounds. The nurses weighed our luggage, and I was asked to get on the scale and the nurses recorded my weight. I tried unsuccessfully to convince the nurses that their scale was wrong and that I weighed over two hundred pounds so that we could bring more belongings with us. They laughed and told me that I was the first person who ever tried that and that they admired my quick thinking. The nurses then recorded Meaghan's weight and her vitals and transferred her care to the escort team. The same triage team that we had met sixteen days earlier was assigned to accompany us. The team was unsure if Jim would be allowed on the tarmac, so we said goodbye at the hospital. We all hugged and cried, uncertain of what lay ahead. I felt like we were heading off to war, and in retrospect we were… against a silent, merciless, and faceless enemy.

The ambulance took us to a private airstrip where we met the pilot and co-pilot. They directed us to a small twin-engine plane on the runway. I thanked both pilots for donating their time and plane to transport Meaghan and then made an off color remark about how size matters, especially with airplanes. Both pilots seemed rather annoyed by my attempt at humor and immediately asked me to find a seat. I don't enjoy flying, and once I factored in the size of the plane, I knew I would need medication, so I reached into my purse, took two motion sickness pills, and hoped to be asleep soon after take-off. The size of the plane did not bother Meaghan at all. She was in a great mood - happy, excited, and hopeful that the answers to her health problems awaited her in Boston.

Once aboard the plane, I was absolutely astounded by the amount of medical equipment that was needed for a medical transport. Only then did I understand the weight restrictions and felt somewhat embarrassed for trying to bring along additional possessions with us. Meaghan was on a stretcher and had tubes and monitors attached to almost every part of her body. She passed the time listening to her iPod and reading a "teen trash" novel for entertainment. The trip was uneventful, save one exception. Meaghan began to have problems blowing out her IV's, and the triage team had to continually find new veins to deliver the medication. Within the hour, we landed at Logan airport in Boston. An ambulance from Children's Hospital was waiting for us on the tarmac.

The triage team escorted us to Boston Children's as they were responsible for Meaghan's care until she was officially transferred to the new hospital. As we wound through the streets of Jim's hometown, Meaghan enjoyed the beauty of the city and was excited about seeing relatives. I did not share in her enthusiasm. I could only think about what was ahead – radiation, chemotherapy, rehab, and possibly another surgery. I smiled as she talked, even though my heart was breaking. I was terrified that we would not get the answer that we were so desperately seeking. I had watched my sister fight cancer for over two years; it is not easy, and neither are the side effects of chemotherapy. I feared for Meaghan, and I feared that I might fail in my care for her.

We arrived at Boston Children's Hospital around noon. Meaghan was immediately taken to the Neuro-Oncology floor. The unit was in the middle of a renovation. The rooms were small, our view was of a roof, and all we could hear were helicopters landing constantly at the medical complex, like something out of *M*A*S*H*. Meaghan and I simultaneously burst into tears. We immediately called Jim, who was on his way to Texas, and blamed him for our current predicament. Almost immediately upon our arrival, family members appeared and laughter filled the room. By the time Jim landed in Texas, Meaghan and I agreed that this is where we needed to be and that we needed to apologize to him for our earlier verbal barrage.

Erin, Jim's niece, came to the hospital that evening. With the help of a floor nurse and two aides, she helped me give Meaghan a bath and wash her hair for the first time since the surgery. Although the steri-

Meaghan's Story

strips still covered the surgical-site, the doctors felt that the wound had healed enough that it was now safe for Meaghan to bathe. The surgical-site was in the back of Meaghan's neck, and because she had been in so much pain, I had not seen the entire scope of her surgery until we went to transfer her to a shower chair. Her scar began about an inch and a half into her hairline and encompassed the entire length of her neck and continued for approximately another two inches into her upper back. I was literally sickened when I saw the extent of her surgery, and I needed to take a moment to collect myself before we continued. Erin, who is an RN, was also taken aback. We just looked at each other with tears in our eyes and shook our heads in disbelief.

It took the five of us over two hours to complete Meaghan's first shower. Since Meaghan was so weak and still in so much pain, we moved her in unison, inches at a time, until we got her into a sitting position at the edge of the bed. Once Meaghan was stable, the others transferred her to a rolling shower chair while I gently supported her back. Then we slowly moved her toward the shower. Once we reached the shower stall, we discovered it was not a roll-in, which meant that we would have to lift Meaghan and the shower chair over the lip of the stall and into the shower. Erin washed Meaghan's hair numerous times because it was so tangled and caked with blood from the surgery. (Even though I had washed it with the dry shampoo at CHKD, I never got it very clean.)

After her shower, Meaghan was smiling from ear to ear and was so happy to be clean. She said it made her feel better, both emotionally and physically. I made a promise to Meaghan that night – from that day on, each and every day, she would get a shower and wash her hair unless it became just too unsafe. I kept that vow until the last few days of her life and was heartbroken when we had to stop.

The next day we met Meaghan's oncologist. He gave us the "Cliffs Notes" version of what the next few days would entail. The most important event was an MRI of Meaghan's brain and spine to ensure that the disease had not spread since the surgery. The idea of the cancer spreading had not previously occurred to either Meaghan or me, and it gave us something to obsess about for the next several days until the MRI was completed and we had the results. Thankfully, the MRI was almost identical to the one that was done at CHKD post-surgery and, more importantly, her brain was free of disease.

Unlike CHKD, where we had gotten used to seeing fewer and fewer doctors and had some degree of solitude, at Boston Children's Hospital, doctors arrived in groups. Each group examined Meaghan and then discussed drug and treatment options related to the specialty of the teaching doctor. Boston Children's is part of Harvard Medical School

Janice Herrity

and, therefore, a huge teaching hospital. The daily rounds resembled a television show… but without all the hot doctors and sexual tension.

Meaghan and I soon learned that:

1. A short white coat meant the individual was either a medical student or intern.

2. A long white coat was a resident.

3. A "fellow" was a resident in training for a specialty.

4. "Real" doctors rarely wore coats and had people follow behind them and write everything down.

We also learned about medical rotation. Within a short amount of time, all of the groups would have new members, and we would continually tell each new group or new person Meaghan's story. This routine became tiresome very quickly, so we would ask each "doctor" what they knew and where they were in their rotation, and I often told the floor residents that Meaghan was not in the mood for another exam. Meaghan hated the constant barrage and often when a doctor would come to check on her, she would pretend to be asleep so the doctor would just check her chart and leave. After they were gone, she would open her eyes, look at me, and say, "Sucker."

We found the doctors at Children's to be exceptional, the residents to be competent, and the medical students were simply students, often with huge egos because they were at Harvard Medical School. After a med student would offer an unsolicited opinion regarding Meaghan's condition, we would just roll our eyes at one another and ignore the advice. We began to dislike many of the interns and residents as they so often missed the mark regarding Meaghan's treatment but were always ready to share their "medical expertise." Rounds began early in the morning and continued often until noon; the privacy we experienced in Norfolk became ancient history, and Meaghan frequently felt like a caged animal at the zoo.

Perhaps the oddest exam came late one evening. Meaghan was sound asleep, and I was awake reading a book. The Neuro-Oncology resident checked Meaghan's chart and asked me some questions. She then informed me that the young lady shadowing her was a medical student and asked if I minded answering her questions. I politely agreed. The medical student asked me a series of simple questions and then asked if she could examine Meaghan. I replied in a sarcastic tone, "Sure, if you can do it without waking her." To my utter disbelief, the med student walked over to Meaghan's bed and began her exam. I looked at the student and said, "Honey, I was joking. There's no way you can exam my daughter without waking her."

Meaghan's Story

The medical student looked at me with complete bewilderment. "Oh," she said, and she and the resident left. Meaghan had awakened while the doctors were in the room but pretended to be asleep to avoid another exam. After they left she said to me, "I thought you had to be smart to get into Harvard." We both started to laugh, and I jumped up and closed the door so the resident and med student wouldn't hear us and come back for a repeat performance.

Each day, Meaghan was making remarkable physical progress. She was lifting both legs, sitting unattended at the edge of the bed, standing in the parallel bars, and was able to roll over. Doctors and therapists were delighted by her progress, and we began to feel hope for the first time in weeks. The doctors continued to order numerous tests on different parts of her body, and the results were promising. Her nervous system was receiving and responding to both voluntary and involuntary cues, but the bad news was that her muscle groups were so weak that they could not always carry out the messages.

As Meaghan continued to improve, the doctors removed the machine that was placed on her legs to prevent blood clots. The machine was not only restrictive but also extremely loud, so we were both grateful to see it gone. Meaghan was moving enough that the doctors felt the anti-embolism stockings would be enough to prevent blood clots. They were hot and ugly, but she didn't mind – it was a sign that she was getting stronger. In fact, Meaghan had made so much progress that the leg braces that were made in Norfolk were now too restrictive for her, and she needed to be fitted for new ones.

Although the general trend was positive, not everything was going in Meaghan's favor. Her arms were covered in bruises from the IV's, and she began to experience constant pain in her left hand, especially in her pinky finger. She continued to have problems with veins "blowing out," and the nurses were having a very difficult time finding a good vein to deliver her medicine, so it was decided that Meaghan needed to be switched to oral medications. Meaghan was delighted to be switched to oral medication as the IV's had been in her left arm for weeks, and they made therapy and her daily life very difficult.

The doctors felt that Meaghan's hand pain was due to the positioning of her arm, because it had been taped to a board for weeks to keep the IV's from popping out with movement. They were certain that once the IV's were removed, her hand pain would slowly go away. However, removing the IV's did not stop the hand pain; it actually increased, and within days Meaghan began to lose mobility in her left hand. The intense hand pain she felt was unremitting, and no one could find a resolution.

Janice Herrity

The doctors theorized that because of the location of the surgery, Meaghan most likely had nerve damage, so they increased the dosage of both Neurontin and morphine and added oral Methadone for breakthrough pain. I remember asking the doctors why Meaghan's hand pain would appear now, weeks after surgery. The answer was that the brain can only process one area of pain at a time. The doctors hypothesized that Meaghan's hand pain had most likely been present all along, and once the intense pain in her legs and neck subsided, her brain could now receive and process the messages from her hands.

Meaghan was then referred to a pain specialist. He was very compassionate and added different pain medications, acupuncture, and massage to help alleviate her pain. The therapies did little to help her and the only real relief that Meaghan could get was from compression. So throughout the day, I filled tube socks with rice, heated the socks in a microwave, and placed them on both sides of Meaghan's left hand to help her ease the pain.

In addition to pain medication every six hours, Meaghan took large doses of the steroid Decadron to contain the tumors. The side effects became increasingly evident. One of the side effects of Decadron is increased appetite, and Meaghan was unable to control her hunger. In addition, the steroids caused Meaghan's once clear skin to break out, her face began to bloat (the medical term is moon face), she became extremely emotional (roid rage), and she gained almost sixty-pounds. Her appearance had changed so radically that she could no longer recognize herself in a mirror. The physical therapists covered the mirrors in the therapy room with towels because Meaghan was so repulsed by her own reflection that she would sob whenever she saw herself. Meaghan hated the steroids and would beg every doctor that examined her to stop them. They all understood her aversion to the drugs, but they all told her the same thing: that the steroids were necessary to both her recovery and containment of the cancer.

Meaghan became increasingly depressed over her appearance, and her clothes no longer fit. Since we were in Boston, a shopping mecca of sorts, I was certain that if I left the hospital I could find shops nearby with cute teenage clothing. The seasons had changed, and because we had been able to bring so little clothing with us, I also needed clothing. I left Meaghan for the first time and went shopping. The hospital area is just that, a hospital area, and the only clothing that I could find within walking distance was at the Harvard Coop Bookstore.

They had a limited selection, but I purchased everything I could find in a variety of sizes and colors. I bought t-shirts, shorts, sweatpants, and sweatshirts, all with the Harvard logo on them. Meaghan and I looked absolutely ridiculous in our matching outfits; we were walking billboards for the Ivy League. Meaghan hated that we were dressed alike and said, "It isn't like my life didn't suck enough. Now I'm dressing like my mother… super." I would taunt her and would tell her how much I liked dressing like a teenager and that once we got home, I hoped we could continue the look. I wasn't being cruel because I would have said the same words if she wasn't sick, and I felt treating her differently was the last thing she needed.

Back in Virginia, the boys were floundering. I called home one day to check messages and learned that TJ had missed school the previous day. I then called the high school to make sure this was not an error. The attendance secretary confirmed that TJ had been absent the day before, but he was at school that day with a note from his older brother explaining his absence. The secretary read me the note. It was signed, James C. Herrity, Legal Guardian.

She asked if this was correct, that Jimmy was now TJ's legal guardian. She knew Jimmy from high school and knew that he was not overly dependable or nurturing and was quite concerned that he was left in charge.

I responded, "Yes, Jimmy is currently TJ's guardian, and sadly that's what our life has turned into." I told her not to worry because a responsible twenty year old would be taking over soon. I spoke with TJ that afternoon and asked why he missed school. He replied that his legal guardian had had a party that lasted until five that morning and he couldn't get to sleep. When he woke up it was the afternoon.

My next call was to TJ's "legal guardian." I informed him of our new policy of no more parties! That night at three a.m., I received a call from Jimmy. He was absolutely hysterical. He said that he had just gotten in and found that one of the dogs had diarrhea, and it was all over the house. He asked me what he should do. I told him to call his dad in Texas, and I hung up. Yep, things were going really well. Fortunately for everyone, Jessica arrived later that week.

Although Children's Hospital was chaotic, Meaghan was very happy there. She loved the nurses and was making great strides daily with her physical recovery. The doctors were doing everything they could to help her regain her life, and we felt hopeful that she would beat both the cancer and the paralysis. When Meaghan was strong enough, we would leave her room to go outside, browse the gift shop, or just walk the floor. As we reentered the world and began to talk to other parents and patients on the neuro-oncology floor, we quickly discovered that we were not alone in this battle. We met many other children, all fighting various forms of cancer, and many more with birth defects. What was most shocking to both Meaghan and me was learning that many of the babies on the floor had been born with cancer – we were horrified that cancer could be present in newborns. As we got to know both the patients and their families, each story that we heard was more horrific than the last. We saw a baby in the room next to ours that appeared to be missing facial bones. It was bone chilling and indescribable. The baby was often without a parent, which is not unusual as often parents have other children at home or have to work to maintain health insurance, keep the lights on, and pay the mortgage. But this baby was never alone. The nurses and aides would sit with the child and rock him for hours.

I met one mother who was just given the news that her daughter's brain tumor was benign and inoperable. The little girl, like Meaghan, would receive chemotherapy and radiation to shrink the tumor. The bad news was that the doctors theorized that her daughter would be blind within a few years. Although the news was difficult, she found consolation in the news that her child would live.

We met one young mother from Albany. She and her child were sent to Boston Children's because her child's condition was rare, and he needed the expertise of a research hospital. She was maybe nineteen, unmarried, and unemployed. Her family was nonexistent, and her boyfriend was a pizza deliveryman who was still in Albany. She and her son came by ambulance and were completely unprepared for a lengthy stay. She had spent the last two months in the ICU with her son prior to being admitted to the neuro-oncology floor. She had little money and few personal belongings, and thankfully, the hospital social workers were providing meal vouchers so she could eat. Her son was about eighteen months old and wore a helmet for protection. He continued to have uncontrollable seizures, even on medication.

We also met people who were there because their child had received the wrong medication or had been the victim of a surgical error. Because of these situations, we learned Lesson VII: Always double check medications, as errors do occur within the medical community. We also began to realize that although Meaghan's situation was dreadful, we were fortunate. We had financial resources and health insurance. Meaghan's brothers were self-sufficient, and I was able to be with Meaghan twenty-four hours a day, seven days a week to assist and advocate for her. Lesson VIII: No one should face a hospital stay without a family member as a support system or as an advocate.

Even though CHKD and the Mayo Clinic had classified Meaghan's tumor as a grade IV GBM, Boston Children's and Dana-Farber wanted to verify the pathology in their lab. We were hopeful that the earlier pathology would be faulty, but unfortunately, the Boston labs gave us the same results.

Meaghan's Story

Once the pathology was confirmed and the doctors were certain that there were no surgical options that they wanted to explore, they began to develop a radiation and chemotherapy plan to attack the cancer. Meaghan was enrolled in a Phase II study that combined radiation and oral chemotherapy (Temozolomide and Lomustine) in the treatment of children with high grade gliomas. The study parameters were that Meaghan would receive forty-two days straight of Temozolomide with concurrent radiation five days a week for six weeks. She would then have a four-week rest period. Every six weeks after that, Meaghan would take a higher dose of Temozolomide for five days and one day of Lomustine. She would repeat this protocol for six cycles. Her chemotherapy was scheduled to end almost a year later, in the spring of 2007. Some of the side effects associated with the drugs were nausea, fatigue, and decreased blood counts (red, white and platelets). The side effects were similar to those of radiation. I could now understand why the oncologist at CHKD felt it was best to hold off on the intensive rehabilitation until Meaghan was stronger.

Jim came to Boston and we met with the oncologist and agreed to enroll Meaghan in the study. We assumed this was the only treatment available for her and wanted the very best treatment that the medical community had to offer. Medical studies have many benefits for the patient: They provide advanced medical treatment and patient care, and they have found cures for many diseases. So we were very hopeful that the medical study in which Meaghan was to participate would be the answer to her illness.

Jim and I had read the information, but we were still in a state of shock. We were not as "on guard" as we would normally be and could have agreed to something that was harmful to Meaghan's health. I credit the oncologist at Children's with sitting us down and explaining the study parameters and what our rights as parents were. He told us that Meaghan would get the same treatment protocol even if we chose not to enroll her in the study, but the hospital would not be able to include her treatment results in their reporting. However, this is not the case with all studies. Each one has unique requirements. Lesson IX: Understand what you are signing when you enroll a loved one in a medical study, and ask questions. Do not feel pressured to sign anything until you are completely aware of what you are signing.

It is imperative to ask the physician if the study is a blind study, meaning that the patient could get a placebo and not the test medication. Frequently the medication in a study will be given to the patient at no cost; this is also an important question to ask. We also learned that there is often a difference between a clinical trial and a medical trial, depending on the research facility. We also learned the difference between the phases of a drug.

Phase I and II drugs are still in the "study stage" and are FDA approved only for research hospitals and facilities. The number of patients receiving the drug is usually small, patients often need to meet specific guidelines to be admitted into the study, and frequently the drug is experimental. A Phase III drug has passed the clinical trial stage and the drug has shown it has significant impact in fighting the disease, and it now can be administered to other patients fighting the same disease outside the constraints of a research hospital. Phase IV drugs have met FDA approval regarding both dosing requirements and long-term side effects. Understanding drug phases and clinical studies was crucial in helping us choose treatment options and hospitals later in our journey

Meaghan had reached a point where, according to the insurance company, she was "not sick enough" to be in a hospital. We were told that she would be moved to a rehabilitation facility next. There are two pediatric rehab hospitals in Boston: Franciscans and Spaulding. The insurance company was pushing Spaulding, so I agreed, and I never even checked Franciscans. Spaulding Rehab is located in the Mass Eye and Ear Institute and connected to Massachusetts General. One of the reasons we chose Boston was that there was proton beam radiation right next door at Mass General.

The discharge planner began the paperwork for the transfer, and we were informed that the radio-oncologist at Children's believed that, due the type and grade of Meaghan's tumor, photon radiation at Brigham and Women's (B&W) was necessary to eradicate both remaining tumors and radiate a larger area to reach any unseen tentacles.

B&W is connected to both Dana-Farber and Children's. That meant that each day, Meaghan would need to be transported across town for the procedure. The discharge planner assured me that both hospitals had checked with our insurance company and there would be no problems with her daily transport. I agreed, and we prepared for our next move. However, the information was incorrect. We did not have a transportation rider and were told that we were financially responsible for Meaghan's transport, which would have run into the tens of thousands of dollars for the next two months. Jim and I told the facility that we weren't paying. It was their mistake and they would have to incur the cost, which they reluctantly did.

Before Meaghan was transferred to Spaulding, she needed to undergo masking and mapping at Brigham & Women's in preparation for radiation. Masking involved making a plastic form fitting mesh mask of Meaghan's face. Once the mask was made, it was labeled with her

Meaghan's Story

name and would be worn for each treatment. The technician explained that the mask would be bolted to the radiation table to keep her head completely still and ensure that the radiation beam reached the intended area.

After masking, Meaghan had radiation mapping. This is where they mapped which areas were to receive radiation and calculated the correct dosage and number of treatments – all while trying to avoid damaging both her nerves and areas of the spinal cord that were cancer free.

This was a long and tough day for Meaghan. The X-Ray technician was not informed that Meaghan was not able to bear weight, and while transferring from her wheelchair, Meaghan began to fall to the ground. Fortunately, I was behind the cement wall and ran and caught her before she hit the floor. Lesson X: Inform the technicians or other hospital personnel of any limits or special circumstances regarding the patient. Do not assume that they know everything about your case.

We then met the radio-oncologist after masking and mapping was completed. She was brilliant and the most compassionate doctor we had encountered thus far in our journey. She explained in great detail that starting May 19th, Meaghan would receive radiation Monday through Friday for the next six weeks. She explained that near the end of treatment, the radiation would become more intensive and would focus on the remaining tumor areas. During the first weeks of her radiation, the beam would be spread out to reach any areas that may have cancer but were not large enough to be seen by the MRI. She then discussed the side effects of radiation and let Meaghan ask questions. The doctor's bedside manner and honesty put Meaghan at ease; she never feared the treatment.

The radio-oncologist then introduced us to the radiation team. They explained all the procedures of radiation, including what not to wear (anything with metallic threads or lettering), and told us that prior to Meaghan's first session, she would need to come back and have a "dry run" to make sure that all of the "bugs" had been worked out.

The staff was wonderful, and Meaghan liked and trusted them immediately. Although B&W is not a pediatric hospital, it is connected to both Boston Children's and Dana-Farber and is part of Harvard Medical Hospitals. Boston Children's Hospital does not have a dedicated radiation facility on site, so pediatric patients needing radiation receive it at B&W.

Meaghan then met the Child Life Specialist. Her job was to help children by play/talk therapy and provide a fun and safe environment while they waited their turn for radiation.

Janice Herrity

It had been nearly one month since Meaghan had her surgery, and we had become immersed in this new world. What amazed me most about Meaghan's illness was that I had taken all of our children's good health for granted, always assuming that childhood cancer was for someone else's child. Never again would I ever be that indifferent about the gift of my children's good health.

Chapter 4 – The Trifecta: Chemo, Rehab, and Radiation

> *In the United States, the incidence of cancer among adolescents and young adults is increasing at a greater rate than any other age group, except those over 65 years.*

By the middle of May, Meaghan was discharged from Boston Children's and moved across town to Spaulding Rehabilitation for Children. The first thing we noticed was how quiet the atmosphere was compared to the ordered chaos of a hospital floor. The unit was small and self-contained with a common dining room, play room, and physical therapy room. There were less than twenty-five patients. Meaghan had a large private room with a magnificent view of both the Boston skyline and Boston harbor. Our plan was to stay at Spaulding until the beginning of July when the first round of chemo and radiation were completed. We would then try to get Meaghan strong enough to come home.

While I was getting us unpacked, one of the nurses came to interview Meaghan to get her perspective on her situation. The first question asked of Meaghan was what she wanted to accomplish with her rehabilitation. Her reply was, "I want to walk out of here." I still remember the nurse telling Meaghan that that was a great goal, but that the purpose of a rehab hospital is to make the patient strong enough to be safe at home.

After the nurse left, Meaghan looked at me with tears in her eyes and said, "Nobody thinks I will be able to walk again."

I replied, "I do and you do, and that's all that matters."

Meaghan wiped her tears and then said, "You're right, these people don't know me. I am going to walk again, and their opinion means absolutely nothing."

Meaghan's goal was simple; she wanted to beat the paralysis and reclaim her life, and nothing was going to stop her. Later that same day, one of the physical therapists came and took Meaghan to the gym. She, too, asked Meaghan what she wanted to accomplish with her physical therapy. Meaghan told her the same thing that she told the nurse earlier, "I want to walk out of here." The therapist explained that they would work each day toward her objective but explained that it would be an uphill battle. Meaghan replied that she was aware of the obstacles and that she was "up for the challenge."

Meaghan's therapy was designed to be low impact due to her overall physical condition and the expected side effects of both chemotherapy and radiation. The rehabilitation plan was designed to rebuild Meaghan's muscle groups slowly, ensuring that the gains she made would be permanent. In order to get her nerves and muscles to respond voluntarily, there was a great deal of repetition involved.

Rehab was not easy; it was very slow, tedious, and regimented, but Meaghan loved it, and she could measure real progress after each session. Each day, she worked on sitting alone, rolling over, pulling up her upper torso, lifting her legs, standing, and moving her feet. The regimen was physically exhausting, but Meaghan excelled. In fact, she made so much progress that the therapists had her leg braces cut back several times because she became strong enough to do much of the work herself.

Meaghan still needed the leg braces to assist her in her daily life. They were hot, heavy, ugly, and often hurt, but they helped her, and she wore them without complaint. The leg braces allowed her to transfer to surfaces without assistance, which was a huge step in both her emotional and physical healing.

Meaghan enjoyed the physical aspect of rehab, but she hated the facility. The emotional journey had taken its toll on her. In a little over a month, Meaghan's life had totally changed. She went from being an active, independent high school student to living in a lockdown unit relearning the first two years of her life. She had been in three hospitals, seen countless medical professionals, had lost all sense of privacy, was taking a myriad of pills, and had her every movement and emotion charted.

Regardless of what the medical personnel thought, I felt that the fact that Meaghan was complaining was a good thing. It showed me she still had fight left in her. I, too, had had enough of life in hospitals, but unlike Meaghan, I was free to come and go as I pleased, and I was not the one doing the intense physical and emotional work. I learned a lot about grief and healing in rehab and often wondered if life had thrown me the curve it had just thrown Meaghan, would I be as strong?

There is something about the nighttime that brings out fears in all of us. There were nights when Meaghan asked me to hold her hand

and to check on her constantly, terrified that she would die in her sleep. I, too, admit to that fear, and that fear never went away, even when things were looking up. Meaghan and I would pray together before bed each night, and never once did she ask to be healed. She prayed for others, never herself. I never asked her reasons, but I truly admired the depth of her faith.

I learned something about myself while in Boston. I had experienced the depth of God's Love before, but I had never truly experienced God's Grace. In fact, a few years before, I was mentoring a young woman at our church, and she asked me to explain Grace, but I could not. I can now – Grace is a quiet inner strength given to you by God that allows you to face the unimaginable with compassion, patience, and love.

Meaghan and I began to socialize with the other children and their families at Spaulding. Once again our eyes were opened to the injustice of life. We saw teenagers with injuries from automobile accidents, children with strokes, cancer patients, children with seizure disorders, infants born addicted to drugs, horrific birth defects, a five year old who had been catatonic for almost a year as a result of an overzealous surgeon, and a twelve year old boy who had been shot in the head over twenty dollars.

We also met a three-year-old girl who had recently been diagnosed with a glioblastomia in her brain. This was her second bout with cancer; she was born with a retinoblastoma and had some other disease that required a feeding tube. Her treatment protocol was different from Meaghan's because her tiny body could not tolerate additional radiation without risking serious side effects. Her mother was acutely aware that her daughter was most likely going to die, yet she chose to live each day to the fullest.

Because of the people we met at both Boston Children's and Spaulding, Meaghan and I learned the most important of all, Lesson XI: Life is a Gift. Live each day with joy in your heart. Love, laugh, and forgive because no one is promised a tomorrow.

Meaghan and I found Spaulding to be both depressing and inspirational. We were amazed that we never knew that this world existed before Meaghan's illness, and I secretly wished I still didn't know about it. At Spaulding, Meaghan realized that there were children far worse off than her. Like Boston Children's, many children did not have a family member with them full time. Meaghan felt lucky to be alive and not alone. She thanked me each day for advocating for her, and she began finding her own voice and began taking control of her own situation. She was growing up before my eyes and becoming a strong young woman;

Janice Herrity

I was very proud. Although I could not feel Meaghan's physical and emotional pain, I could only imagine its intensity and marveled at both her strength and her tenacity.

Meaghan and I had always had a very good relationship, but our new world made us especially close. Our bond was unbreakable. In order to survive, we insulated ourselves from the outside world, became best friends, and filled our days with laughter, inside jokes, girl talk, and reality television. I would often think of our journey and compare it to fighting a war. I believe we bonded as men do in battle. The world we were living in was very much a battle: the enemy was cancer, the battlefield was her body, and the goal was to defeat the enemy and to return home alive and in one piece.

Life continued, but it felt as if it stood still for us. Meaghan's routine was exhausting. She woke up at seven-thirty, ate breakfast, and dressed. Physical therapy was at nine, and occupational therapy was at ten. She then rested for an hour, ate lunch, left for radiation, waited her turn for radiation, and endured radiation for fifteen minutes. She would then return to Spaulding, eat dinner, shower, check snail mail and email, watch some reality TV, have a snack, go through chemo, and finally go to bed.

Meaghan's radiation was at Brigham and Women's Hospital, which was approximately four miles away from Spaulding, but due to Boston traffic, it took over an hour to get there most days. Along the route, we passed Fenway Park, and if the Yankees were in town to play the Red Sox, the trip could easily take two hours each way, but Meaghan went each day without complaint.

The insurance company mandated weekly outings in addition to therapy, radiation, and chemo. Meaghan loved these. These included assisted kayaking on the Charles River, shopping, museum visits, and outdoor group activities. In addition, every Wednesday we spent the afternoon at the Jimmy Fund, the children's oncology clinic at Dana-Farber, to have Meaghan's blood work done and see the oncologist.

The pace, coupled with the hot sun, chemo, radiation, and physical therapy began to take its toll on Meaghan's body. One afternoon after a morning outing in Boston, she became too weak to get on to the radiation table. Meaghan was immediately sent to the ER at Children's, and an MRI was ordered. Unbelievably, the scan showed tumor progression, and Meaghan was immediately readmitted back to Children's. (This scenario was unusual as scans are rarely done during radiation.)

I looked at the MRI with the resident and saw that the tumor area was indeed larger and that there was a previously undetected third

Meaghan's Story

tumor. Totally shocked and heartbroken, I called Jim who was in Texas and told him the results; he, too, was in utter disbelief. We had promised Meaghan in Norfolk that we would never hide anything from her, so my next job was to deliver the horrifying MRI results to her.

As I began to search for the words to tell Meaghan that her scan showed disease progression, a neurosurgeon appeared and thankfully interrupted me. He told us that her MRI looked good and that he had no intention of operating. He said that the scans look worse during radiation because of the interaction between the tumor and the radiation. He further explained that the tumor was larger because tumors "often blow up" during radiation and that the third tumor was most likely a tentacle that had gone unseen earlier because it was too small to be detected by the previous MRI's. He apologized for the misinformation and explained that residents do not always have the expertise to read and interpret scans, especially in rare cases - the same lesson that we learned at CHKD a month earlier.

The oncologist and radio-oncologist felt that even though Meaghan's scans looked good, she should be re-admitted to Children's for observation and, hopefully, to get some badly needed rest.

In the meantime, the oncology fellow increased Meaghan's Decadron dosage without informing either Meaghan or me. Meaghan had been on steroids since the ICU and was days from being weaned off them. (Due to the nature of the drug and her dosage, a slow wean was needed.) Meaghan hated the steroids, and the new dosage was so large that it would take at least another month before she would be completely weaned off steroids once more.

I was so angry with that "Doctor" that I had her paged to Meaghan's room and explained in no uncertain terms that her decision was reckless and unwarranted and that it was completely unprofessional to prescribe a drug without consulting the patient or the parent! I also told her that that I would be requesting that she be removed from Meaghan's case immediately. If she were the only physician on the floor and Meaghan had a problem, she should call someone else. She was not to go anywhere near my daughter. I also informed her that she was very lucky because I was "just too damn tired to pursue legal action" against her. From that day forward, both Meaghan and I questioned everything a resident or fellow did regarding her treatment. We became very annoyed at the continued lack of respect that many had for their patients.

That evening Meaghan needed her chemotherapy, which was back at Spaulding. Thankfully, Erin volunteered to go pick it up for me so I didn't have to leave Meaghan. Once Erin got to Spaulding, she was informed that she needed to take all of our belongings with her, because Meaghan had to be discharged from Spaulding before she could be admitted to Boston Children's.

We spent the weekend at Children's, and on Monday, Meaghan was readmitted to Spaulding, so we had to haul all of our possessions back across town. Once Meaghan was readmitted, Spaulding was required to do a physical reevaluation to comply with insurance, even though she was gone for only a few days.

Meaghan learned that she was totally helpless in her new world. The insurance company and doctors controlled her world, and she developed, for lack of a better description, a "Stockholm Syndrome" personality around health professionals in order to survive. She had learned that if she cried or complained about her predicament that a child life specialist, psychologist, or a psychiatrist was sent to talk with her.

Meaghan learned to manipulate her therapists and would look at them and say, "If you were me, wouldn't you cry? Wouldn't you be angry if you lost your independence? Wouldn't you be pissed if you had to relearn the first two years of your life? How would you like to live in a lockdown unit and have every second of your life recorded?"

Once she turned the questions and emotions on her therapists, the sessions often ended. I was very proud of her ability to advocate for herself. I saw it as a positive and healthy sign that she was adjusting psychologically to her situation. But we were both sure that her medical chart showed just the opposite!

Back in Virginia, my friends and Jessica were packing up the old house and preparing it for sale, as well as getting things ready in the new house for our return. It was my job to renovate the new house and make it handicap accessible. Living in a rehab facility made me acutely aware that major changes would be needed to make Meaghan's transition to home easier. Our new house had carpet throughout, which needed to be replaced with laminate flooring. Interior doors needed to be enlarged to accommodate a wheelchair, either through door extensions or by enlarging the opening. We needed to find a way to get Meaghan in and out of the house either with a ramp or a lift, and we needed to purchase and replicate much of the rehab equipment Meaghan was using at Spaulding to make daily life less problematic for her.

Even though our new house was a ranch, there was a room upstairs that Meaghan had chosen prior to her illness. We were determined that she was coming home to that room, so we needed to install a stair lift to the second floor. I was adamant that Meaghan would be able to maneuver with ease in our new home. The only rooms that were not made handicap accessible were the boy's bedrooms and bath - simply because we ran out of money.

The renovations and medical equipment were costly, and most were not covered by insurance, so we did what most people would do in this situation, we reached for the credit card. Within a short time, we had exhausted our savings account and were tens of thousands of dollars in debt. Then the medical bills arrived, and we had no money to pay them so they, too, went on the credit card.

Little by little the overwhelming obstacles were lessening, but as always there were unforeseen challenges ahead. Each day, Meaghan was getting stronger and needed less and less assistance. She was surprising doctors and therapists alike with her physical recovery, and they all began to believe that she would soon walk again.

She continued to experience recurrent bladder and kidney infections, and her hand pain at times became unbearable. The doctors and therapists at both Spaulding and Children's tried every therapy they could think of to lessen her pain. They tried acupuncture, nerve blocks, nerve distraction, electrical stimulation, heat, ice, and compression, but the only relief Meaghan could get was from an isotoner glove.

A doctor at Children's referred Meaghan to a pain specialist who was in private practice. Because of the referral, we were able to see the doctor the following day. Meaghan's schedule was extremely tight the day of the appointment because she needed to be across town for her weekly appointment at the Jimmy Fund, and she had radiation after that. We waited a very long time to see the doctor, but we didn't mind because both Meaghan and I were hopeful that this doctor would have the answer to Meaghan's hand pain.

The specialist quickly examined Meaghan and then told her that much of her pain was in her head and that she needed to work on distracting herself from it, perhaps "imagining herself on a beach." The doctor then handed me her card and instructed me to make a follow-up appointment in two weeks. I looked at her and said, "No, Thank you, we will not need your services" and handed her card back to her. I wanted to tell her what I really thought of her, but she was referred by another physician that we respected, so I said nothing. I had learned from our experience with interns and residents that the medical community sticks together. I am convinced it is an unspoken oath they take when they become doctors, but of course I can't get anyone to admit to it!

Even as I write this over three years later, I am still incensed by that doctor's arrogance and dismissive nature. Meaghan had major surgery on her central nervous system, tumors still remained in her spinal cord and this broad insisted Meaghan's pain was all in her head!

Janice Herrity

Jim was working in Texas so on weekends he split his time between Boston and Virginia, trying to keep in touch with the boys and see Meaghan as much as possible. (He said there were times he would get to George Bush Airport in Houston and have to look at his ticket, because he had no idea where he was going.)

On weekends, Meaghan was allowed to leave Spaulding as long as she was not gone for more than twenty-four hours, otherwise per insurance she would have had to been discharged. Jim and I would take Meaghan around Boston and it really helped her mental and emotional psyche to get away from the confinement of a hospital.

We often walked to Faneuil Market or to Cambridge, or just sat by the Charles River and watched the boats. Many of Boston's streets are cobblestone, making the pavement very uneven, which made it very difficult for us to maneuver Meaghan in a wheelchair, let alone her push herself. We also discovered that not every shop was wheelchair accessible, or that the displays were often so crowded together that Meaghan could not go down aisles, stalls in bathrooms were used by the non-handicapped population leaving Meaghan to wait, and in one store we found the handicap dressing room stacked with boxes of merchandise waiting to be processed so Meaghan could not try on clothing. We then learned Lesson XII: The world is not handicap accessible.

When Meaghan became strong enough to take day trips in a car, parking became an issue. We began to notice the number of people who seemed to abuse handicap parking. Many used a placard because of its convenience, not because they were truly disabled. (I do know that many people with placards have disabilities that cannot be "seen," and I want to acknowledge that I am not diminishing their disability. They are entitled to the placards, but there is a great deal of abuse in the system.) Frequently, groups would walk right in front of Meaghan and crowd in front of her in elevators. Individuals often stared or turned their heads to avoid eye contact. This made her feel invisible. She would look at us with tears in her eyes and say, "They don't see me; they only see a girl in a wheelchair." Jim and I were outraged by Meaghan's treatment and would often express our anger verbally to the offenders. This embarrassed Meaghan, so we learned to just keep quiet and let the anger seethe. We then learned Lesson XIII: Anger is counter-productive. We needed to adjust to Meaghan's new world without anger or bitterness; otherwise we would hinder her recovery.

Back home, we were scheduled to move on June 15th. Offers from friends wanting to help poured in. Jessica, Kim, and Julia coordinated the move, so Jim could focus on work. They packed the house and labeled each and every box and then called me and told me what a boring life

Meaghan's Story

I led – there was no porn, no sex toys - nothing except tons of school supplies, batteries, candles, and paper products.

Jimmy and Jessica took a walk through the new house and decided everything was fine. They had no idea what they were doing or what to look for, but they signed off so the renters could have their deposit back. In retrospect, I cannot believe that we had two twenty-year olds handle our real estate transaction, but we had no other choice.

Jessica took phone calls and made herself available to let the workmen into the new house so they could get as much done prior to the move as possible. Meaghan's room was the priority, so that's where the work began. The carpet was ripped out, and laminate flooring was installed. Then her room was painted a new color. Meaghan's room had a private bath, but the entrance was awkward so it was relocated and enlarged to accommodate a wheelchair, which involved repositioning much of the existing plumbing and wiring. The bathroom vanity was removed and replaced with a pedestal sink, and grab bars were installed on the bathroom walls and in the bathtub for safety. We also enlarged the opening to the half bath downstairs and made it handicap accessible to allow Meaghan privacy on the first floor.

We were told that Meaghan's illness entitled her to a wish through the Make-A-Wish Foundation, but we were very reluctant to accept, because we had heard that the wishes were only for children who were likely to die within a short period of time. The volunteers assured us that this was a common misconception and encouraged us to let them grant Meaghan "A Wish." Since Meaghan wanted her wish, we relented. For her wish, Meaghan chose a bedroom make over. She found the perfect items on Target's website, emailed them to the volunteers in Virginia, and together they planned her new room. I was still very hesitant about accepting the wish and told Meaghan not to be too excessive in her choices and to always keep the cost of the items in mind, which she gladly did. However, Make-A-Wish was very generous and in addition to the bedspread and curtains Meaghan requested, they purchased a canopy bed, dresser, bookcases, bedside table, pictures, knick-knacks, and a rocking chair – all in the "shabby chic" theme Meaghan chose. The Make a Wish volunteers were absolutely wonderful and worked diligently to finish Meaghan's room prior to our return home.

Jim came home for the move and was amazed by the number of people (many of whom he had never met before) who had showed up to help. Because there was an abundance of volunteers, it took less than two hours to move all of our belongings to our new home. Once everything was there, the volunteers began to unpack the boxes and put things away.

Janice Herrity

Karen and my brother-in-law drove up from North Carolina to help as well. Karen had chemotherapy earlier in the week and was still very sick from the effects of the drugs, but she insisted on assisting. I had told my sister that the only rooms I wanted completed before we returned from Boston were Meaghan's room and the kitchen, so that's where they began. Karen arranged my collection of baskets on the soffit above the cupboards and displayed my knickknacks. Friends unpacked and washed all of our pots, pans, glasses, utensils, and dishes and then lined the cupboards. One of my girlfriends had noticed that the cupboards were lined at our old house and decided that since I am anal retentive, I must like my cupboards lined. She went out and bought the same shelf paper that I had at my old house to ease my transition home. Unbeknownst to her, it had taken me ten years to line the cupboards of the old house, so this was a bonus… and perhaps I was not as obsessive-compulsive as she thought! The next week, Jessica, Kim, Julia, and numerous friends began to prepare the old house for sale by patching holes and painting walls.

Within days of moving into to the new house, the air conditioning condenser broke and had to be replaced. Bees built a hive under the deck and were swarming at anyone who went near them. TJ had a car accident and passed out at school. The lawn mower caught fire, and when Jimmy purchased a new one, it, too, was defective. The flooring for the downstairs was delayed, so the floors would not be installed in most of the house before we returned. Lola, one of our dogs, developed an infection that required antibiotics and eventually surgery. The old house smelled of dogs and required numerous carpet and professional cleanings, and lastly, the real estate market had cooled and selling the house was going to be harder and less lucrative than we had anticipated.

Back in Boston, radiation and chemo were to be finished by the end of June. Although it would have been a good idea to stay and continue rehab, both Meaghan and I were ready to go home. Meaghan had been pushed to her emotional limits, and she was tired of crappy food, lack of privacy, and the controlled atmosphere of a hospital. I, too, was ready to leave. I had not slept in a real bed for months. I slept in a chair that pulled out to a hard, small bed. Each night when I converted the chair to a bed, I would cover the chair deck with pillows and create a makeshift mattress and then put a fitted sheet over the pillows to keep them in place. It was not comfortable, but I was so grateful that I could stay with Meaghan that I would have slept on the floor. Meaghan and I had spent seventy-eight straight days in hospitals, and we were counting down the days until she was to be discharged.

Luckily, Meaghan never got as sick from the chemo and radiation as the doctors predicted. The only real side effects that she experienced were thrush and a bad sunburn on the back of her neck from the

Meaghan's Story

radiation, along with nausea and some vomiting from the chemotherapy. I was truly amazed at how well she had handled the difficult regimen and very proud of how she matured through the adversity.

I was also relieved that I had trusted my maternal instincts as opposed to the advice from doctors and insisted that Meaghan receive rehab at the same time as chemo and radiation. I often think back and cannot believe what I put that girl through. I am not sure if I truly knew the intensity of the treatments that I would have pushed for the chemo, radiation, and rehab at the same time.

Although radiation was considered to be hard on the body, Meaghan enjoyed going. She made numerous CD's to listen to while getting her treatment. Since radiation, for the most part, is passive, Meaghan could relax. Since her treatment was considered outpatient, the atmosphere at B&W was less controlled. Unlike Spaulding's and Children's Hospital that blocked certain websites like MySpace and Facebook, B&W allowed unrestricted internet access, Meaghan could chat online with friends while she waited her turn for radiation

We met many children and their families in the pediatric waiting room, each fighting cancer, all with very different diagnosis. No one pitied himself or herself, and no one complained. I was always awed by the courage and bravery of these children. On occasion, I would wait in the adult area, and the atmosphere was completely different from the children's room. Patients were full of fear, self-pity, and anger and they grew impatient if the technicians were running behind. (As if you would want a technician to rush through your radiation!)

One day I was in the adult area waiting for Meaghan to finish her radiation and began to chat with a man sitting across from me. He was in his mid-sixties and told me that he was waiting his turn for radiation and that he had prostate cancer. After our brief conversation, he returned to his newspaper, and I began to read my book. He must have forgotten where he was because at some point he uncrossed his legs and exposed his "man junk." After Meaghan finished her treatment I told her that I made a new friend in the waiting area, and that he "flashed" me. I told her that perhaps tomorrow she could wait with me and with any luck there would be a repeat performance. She just rolled her eyes and said, "eww gross" and told me that she had enough friends.

As I mentioned before, the steroids caused Meaghan to gain nearly sixty pounds. As a consequence, her radiation mask no longer fit comfortably. Radiation had gone very smoothly and Meaghan had no problems with the routine until the last day, when her mask became so tight from her weight gain that once the techs bolted it to the table it began to cut off her air supply. Meaghan said that in the middle of the

Janice Herrity

session she began to have difficulty breathing and then began to black out. She said that her CD was blaring and the techs were behind the wall, so they were unaware she was having a problem. To get their attention, she began to frail her arms and legs wildly.

The technicians stopped the beam and ran to Meaghan's aid. They saw that she was gasping for air, unbolted her mask from the table, sat her up, and discussed suspending her radiation until a new mask could be made for her final treatment. Meaghan told the technicians to proceed and said that she was determined to finish her radiation that day. She told the techs that she would deal with the discomfort and assured them she would be fine but reminded them to keep their eyes on her in case the problem occurred again. She also said that she had no intention of letting her legacy be that she was the girl who was choked to death by her mask on her last day of radiation.

They proceeded, and she finished her last treatment. When Meaghan came out to the waiting area I could see that the mask had left a crisscross impression across her face, and the techs told me what happened. I just looked at them and burst out laughing because radiation had gone so easily that, of course, Meaghan would have a problem on her last day. It was just her luck.

Prior to leaving rehab, Meaghan was determined that she was going to walk, and with the assistance of two physical therapists (one holding her hip and the other placing her feet) Meaghan walked nineteen feet straight on a walker. All the children in the unit were watching and cheering her on; it was truly a magical moment. Meaghan was absolutely exhausted afterward, but she walked. I attribute her success to a positive attitude, hard work, and inner strength. Although Meaghan did not walk out of rehab as she had hoped, she was walking with a walker, transferring to surfaces alone, rolling over, and sitting unassisted for long periods of time – in short, she beat the odds.

We said our goodbyes to the family, friends, therapists, nurses, and doctors who had contributed to Meaghan's success and packed up for a commercial flight home as Meaghan was strong enough that an air ambulance was no longer needed. Jim flew to Boston to accompany us. Erin and her fiancée drove the majority of our belongings (mostly from the Harvard Coop) back to Virginia and met us later that day. We had come to Boston a little over two months earlier with one bag each, and it now took a van to move us home. Thank you, retail therapy!

Chapter 5 – Be It Ever So Humble, There's No Place Like Home

> *Childhood cancers are the #1 disease killer of children - more than asthma, cystic fibrosis, diabetes, and pediatric AIDS combined.*

Once we arrived at Logan Airport, we checked our bags and continued on to security. Meaghan was not ambulatory, so she could not be screened through the standard security lines. A female TSA agent took her to a private area for screening. Jim and I were instructed that we could not accompany Meaghan, but once we cleared security, we could then enter the TSA private screening area to get her and proceed to our gate.

After about ten minutes we cleared security and went to find Meaghan. Once we entered the secure area, we could see that she was still with the TSA agent, visually upset, and fighting back tears. The TSA agent had asked Meaghan for her photo identification, and she replied that she didn't have one with her. The agent then told her that she could not clear security because Transportation Safety Administration policy dictates that travelers must have some form of photo identification in order to enter the restricted area of the airport and board their flight. The agent then asked us for Meaghan's photo ID, and we replied that the only things that we had with us to identify her as Meaghan Herrity were her medication and numerous prescriptions to fill once we got home.

I showed them to the agent, and she just looked at me and then explained in great detail the TSA regulations regarding photo ID's. Meaghan burst into tears, absolutely petrified that she wouldn't be able to board the plane.

Traveling is part of Jim's weekly routine, so he knew instinctively that this situation wasn't going to rectify itself, so he went and found the agent's supervisor. Jim explained that Meaghan had been transported by air ambulance directly from the hospital in Norfolk to Boston Children's and amid everything that was happening in our lives, it never occurred to us to bring along a photo ID for Meaghan. Thankfully, the supervisor was very understanding and let us proceed to our gate.

Janice Herrity

Due to Meaghan's health, we were able to board the plane early. We purchased first class tickets to make sure that Meaghan would have plenty of space to enter and exit the rows. Since Meaghan's wheelchair was too large to navigate the narrow airplane aisles, we needed to transfer her to a special wheelchair designed specifically for use in airplanes. Jim and I, along with the airline personnel, helped Meaghan transfer to a small wheelchair and then belted her in for safety, maneuvered her through the aisle, and transferred her to her seat.

Once we got Meaghan settled, she began to read a book, and I took full advantage of the benefits of first class. I ordered a cocktail and then drank two more before we were cleared for takeoff. I continued to reap the benefits of first-class until I had to give up my drink as we prepared for landing in Newport News.

Although I was not the patient, living in hospitals had drained me mentally and emotionally, but the effects were much more profound for Meaghan. The constant scrutiny of medical personnel, the scope of her treatments, the loss of her independence, and the extent of her overall physical situation had taken a toll on her psyche. I had witnessed Meaghan mature, but I had also seen her pushed to her emotional limits. I vowed to myself that we would never put her through another extensive hospital stay again unless it was absolutely medically necessary.

The flight from Boston was uneventful, and we arrived in Newport-News around 1:30 in the afternoon. Meaghan was the last to leave the airplane because we once again had to use the special wheelchair to get her through the narrow aisle and off the airplane. We then transferred Meaghan to her regular wheelchair, which we brought with us and kept in the main cabin of the aircraft. Jim went to collect our baggage, and Meaghan and I met Jessica and the boys in the loading zone in front of the airport.

The trip from Boston and the summer heat had left Meaghan so weak that it took four of us to get her from the wheelchair into the car. Once she was safely inside, Jimmy and TJ pulled me aside and asked me what had happened to her. Meaghan's appearance had changed so drastically as a result of the steroids that her brothers barely recognized her. She no longer resembled the sister that left for Boston two months earlier.

As we drove onto our street, we could see our new house in the distance. It was decorated with "Welcome Home Meaghan" signs. Jimmy told Meaghan that several of her friends had come over earlier that day, decorated the house, brought her cookies, and wanted to be there when she arrived. Meaghan became very agitated and said that she hoped that her friends were not waiting at the house because she was embarrassed by

Meaghan's Story

her appearance and that once they saw her, they would only pity her. It was only then that I realized that her scars were more than just physical and that reentering the world was going to be quite difficult.

Once we got to our new home, our first challenge was getting Meaghan out of the car and into the house. We had installed a stair lift in the garage to go up the three steps to the laundry room and then once inside, we needed to maneuver her into the main living area. When I was planning out the modifications for the house, it never occurred to me that Meaghan would not be strong enough to do the transfer herself or that she would require assistance to use the stair lifts. Since I was the only one that was trained in lifting and that knew her physical limitations, getting her safely into the house fell upon my "expertise."

I examined the situation, formulated a plan, and then "crossed my fingers." Getting Meaghan into the house would mean transferring her from the car to her wheelchair and lifting her onto the stair lift. We would then run her wheelchair back through the garage, up the front steps through the front door, then through the house to the laundry room and lift Meaghan off the lift and finally transfer her to the wheelchair. Once we got Meaghan inside the laundry room, we hit another obstacle. The dryer blocked the stair lift, so we had to move the washer and dryer, along with a cabinet, to make room for her wheelchair. It took all five of us working together, but we got Meaghan safely into the house.

Once inside, Meaghan was anxious to see her room, so we transferred her to the stair lift that would take her to the second floor. Because we had never lived in the house, I remembered the landing at the top of the stairs as larger than it actually was and planned the modifications for a more spacious area. Due to the limited size of the landing at the top of the staircase, the transfer off the stair lift became both complicated and dangerous. Meaghan was insistent that she see her new room, so we devised a plan that would keep Meaghan from falling down the stairs in case the transfer went poorly and we dropped her. Jimmy and Jessica blocked the top of the staircase with their bodies, TJ held the wheelchair in place, and Jim and I lifted Meaghan off the stair lift and into the wheelchair.

Make-A-Wish had done a wonderful job decorating her room. It looked exactly as she had planned. Meaghan was overjoyed with the final result, and once she finished touring her room, the five of us lifted her into her bed. After Meaghan was safely in bed, we let the dogs in the house. They immediately jumped on Meaghan's bed and cuddled next to her. I believe that at that moment she began to heal emotionally.

The first few days home were absolutely insane. There were still many moving boxes that needed to be unpacked, and cartons of laminate flooring were stacked in hallways. The bees returned, and the weight of both Jim's and my clothing ripped the rods from the master closet, so our clothing lay in a pile on the floor. The previous owners had not properly deactivated the security system, and somehow it was set off at one in the morning.

Meaghan's nervous system was still incredibly sensitive from the operation. She had a great deal of difficulty adjusting to noise, and she had not yet regained the ability to filter out background sounds. The blaring siren was causing her to shriek in pain. We didn't know the shut off code, so we had to call the sheriff to stop the piercing alarm noise. Since we did not have a phone number for the alarm company or an access code, the sheriff, with my blessing, ripped the box off the wall and tossed the control panel into the garage.

The lawnmower caught fire. The boys went to purchase a new one only to find that it, too, was defective. They purchased yet another, and it had a fuel line problem. (We went through four lawn mowers in over a month, if you were keeping count.) Completely exasperated, we called a friend that was a mechanic, and he fixed the problem so the boys could mow the lawns at both houses.

The housing market had slowed, so we were having difficulty selling our old house and of course had two mortgage payments and two sets of utility bills. Our cable television and phone service stopped working due to a technical glitch that was in some way related to the number of televisions and computers we had in use. Almost daily I would call the cable company and go through the series of automated options until I reached a human being, tell my story, and then schedule service. Because I was on hold so often I learned how to pass the artificial intelligence by making random babbling sounds when the system would ask a question. Without fail I would be immediately connected to a human and plead for help. (By the way, this only works between the hours of nine and five, Monday through Friday.) The situation continued for several weeks until one day I broke down sobbing and was passed to a "special customer service unit." They took pity on me and sent someone who worked exclusively with their unit to our home to fix the problem. This may sound odd, but the only problem that caused me to crack was the lack of cable TV and internet. I think it was either the final straw or the frustration that such a simple problem took so much time and effort that I needed to direct elsewhere.

Little by little, life slowed down, and we developed a daily routine. Jim returned to Texas, and Jessica stayed until mid-July to help us settle in. Meaghan was still having difficulty sitting up for long periods of time and was still very weak. We decided that she needed a hospital bed until she was stronger, so we had one brought in and placed in the

Meaghan's Story

master bedroom. Although Meaghan wanted to be in her room, she was still so weak that having her near me was a good thing.

Our next dilemma was that the only handicap accessible bathroom was upstairs. We needed to figure out a way for Meaghan to bathe safely downstairs. The boy's bathroom door was not large enough for a wheelchair, and the master bath had a soaking tub and separate glass shower. We tried the soaking tub but soon discovered that it was just too unsafe, so we removed the glass doors from the shower and placed a shower bench inside. We soaked the bathroom every time she showered, but it was safer than having her go upstairs and risk injury. The insurance company would pay for the rental on her wheelchair, minus our monthly co-pay, but we soon learned that we needed three wheelchairs to make life easier for us – one in the car, one on the first floor, and one on the second, so we purchased two more chairs.

We also found it necessary to duplicate other medical equipment and would spend close to twenty-five thousand dollars that summer in additional modifications to our house to make Meaghan's life easier.

Life didn't quiet down entirely. TJ was sort of carjacked/kidnapped while helping a stranger at the mall. He had gone to purchase a video game and called Meaghan as he was leaving and asked her if she wanted ice cream. It was over ninety degrees, and Meaghan thought the ice-cream would be melted by the time he reached home, so she declined. He then told her that he'd be right home so they could play the game. About forty-five minutes later, Meaghan became concerned that something had happened to him and suggested that I call him to see if he was okay because the mall was only a ten minute drive, even in congested traffic.

I called, and TJ answered, but all I could hear was a woman in the background yelling. I asked if the voice was a police officer and he replied, "No, it was some woman who came to my car asking for money, and when I wouldn't give her any, she began to pass out and climbed into the car." I still am unsure how she got control of the keys, but she was driving and they were en route to Norfolk. I called the Hampton police, told them the story, gave them a description of the car, and they said that they would do what they could.

In the interim, Meaghan called Jimmy to see if he could help and then he in turn called TJ's cell and asked to speak to the woman. He told her that he was "armed" and had the car in view so she had better pull over. They were stopped in traffic near the Hampton Roads Bridge Tunnel, and she immediately jumped out of TJ's car and got into a car behind them and took off. TJ took possession of the car and called me to say he was okay. (Jimmy was actually working, but his rouse worked.)

Janice Herrity

I called my friend, Kim, to stay with Meaghan so I could go assist TJ, but Meaghan was adamant that she was coming along. Since I was in no mood to argue with her, I agreed. I got Meaghan out of bed, into the wheelchair, on to the stair lift, off the lift, into the wheelchair, and into the car without help from anyone. We were both so proud of ourselves because it was a coordinated effort, and, more importantly, Meaghan was now strong enough to assist.

We picked up Kim and then headed to Hampton to find TJ. Once we reached TJ, and I found out that he was okay, I talked to the police. They informed me that this was a scam used by "gangs and crack heads" on young kids that were alone. They most likely were going to "roll him," keep the car, and abandon him in downtown Norfolk. TJ was clearly stunned by what the policeman told him. He looked at me and said it never occurred to him that this woman could have done him serious harm.

I had Kim drive Meaghan home, and I went with TJ. He kept apologizing and felt horrible that Meaghan had to leave the house. I told him it was no big deal; she wanted to come along, and anyone could have been this woman's victim. I told him to shake it off and learn from the experience. If by chance it ever happened again, he should get out of the car and let the crack-head keep it. I then told him the good news – that we got out of the house by ourselves. There was a silver lining: he was okay, and Meaghan and I did the car transfer without assistance from anyone.

Meaghan began out-patient rehab within a week of returning home. We chose not to go to CHKD but to a local hospital as her body was the size of an adult, and she was tired of seeing so many sick kids. I admit that I was, too. My heart and psyche needed a break from all the childhood sickness we had witnessed over the last three months. The hospital was not in our insurance network, so we were responsible for thirty percent of the charges. Since we were so used to hemorrhaging money, it became a non-issue, and we just accepted the situation and wrote the check each time she had therapy.

Meaghan's first session was July sixth. Before the therapists could develop a treatment plan, they needed to do an assessment of Meaghan's physical condition. This involved a series of motor tests to determine her baseline. Our first appointment was with the occupational therapist. He did his evaluation and then listened to Meaghan as she talked about her incessant hand pain. The operation, radiation, and remaining tumors in her spinal cord had left her peripheral nervous system garbling messages, and she experienced constant neuropathy. Meaghan described the neuropathy as "pins and needle pain" that intensified with touch.

Meaghan's Story

The occupational therapist (OT) immediately began working on desensitizing Meaghan's hands and fingertips against the neuropathy by placing her hands in an enclosed machine with cornhusks that whirled around a container heated by air. He then began to massage the area and get her hands and fingertips used to external stimuli. By the time our session was complete, Meaghan had her first relief from hand pain in months! She was ecstatic, and we were both astonished that even though she had been in some of the best hospitals in the world, we had not seen this machine before. The OT explained that this was not unusual as the machine is mostly used in outpatient treatment and not in a hospital setting. Lesson XIV: The outpatient world of a hospital operates much differently than the inpatient world. The OT explained that the procedures and equipment in an outpatient setting are geared for patients needing more intensive rehabilitation than in a hospital setting.

We also learned that the therapists would need to document Meaghan's treatment and progress each month and that they must get approval from the insurance company for additional visits. The therapist's would have to show that additional therapy was medically necessary to have our insurance company pay for rehabilitation. I had learned early on in our journey that health care is a business, and if the patient does not show improvement, insurance payments will be suspended. If the patient continued treatment, they would be responsible for services out of pocket. Jim and I were prepared to do this, but fortunately it never became an issue.

Our next appointment was with the physical therapist (PT). He, too, did an evaluation, followed by exercises to strengthen both Meaghan's legs and trunk, and then said to her, "Let's do some walking." Meaghan and I looked at each other like he was crazy. She had walked only once before, with help from a therapist holding her hip and another assisting with her foot placement. Meaghan was worried about falling, but the PT assured her that he would be right beside her, and a PT associate would follow her with a wheelchair should she become tired and need to sit down.

The therapist took Meaghan out into the hallway in her wheelchair, placed a physical therapy safety belt around her waist, and helped her stand. Once she was stable, she began to place one foot in front of the other and walked with a walker twenty-two feet unassisted!! It took every bit of strength Meaghan could muster, and she was absolutely exhausted afterward, but she walked unassisted!

Jessica and I stood there with tears of joy streaming down our faces, and Meaghan was smiling from ear to ear. She then told the therapist, "Next time I come for therapy, I will walk twenty-five feet!" When she came back later that week, she walked thirty.

The first month home, Meaghan was on a rest period from chemotherapy, so she was strong enough for physical and occupational therapy three times a week. She quickly connected with her therapists, and friendships developed. Her work ethic, together with her personality, made her a favorite of the therapists. She would act as if she was going to fall every time their supervisor walked by, because she learned that there was a mountain of paperwork involved if someone fell or was injured during a session. Then she would laugh hysterically after the supervisor left.

With each session, the therapists continued to push her body, strengthening her muscles. By the end of July, Meaghan was walking a hundred feet straight in a walker without needing to rest. Her physical therapy consisted of a series of exercises and repetitive movements that would help her regain her physical losses and get her walking independently. The exercises included core strengthening and rebuilding muscle and muscle memory.

The therapists designed a therapy routine that included mat work to strengthen Meaghan's upper body followed by weight work that built and strengthened her leg muscles. She would then stand in the parallel bars to work on coordination and finally climbing stairs and walk. The routine was hard, but she loved going, and each day she was making real progress toward regaining her independence.

Meaghan learned a great deal about herself that month. She learned that "real strength" comes from within and that the greatest obstacle in life is a negative attitude. Although the once stylish Meaghan now wore thigh high anti-embolism stockings, leg braces, and an isotoner glove, she always had a smile on her face and a positive attitude, and she accepted her situation with a quiet grace. Even though Meaghan's body was broken, her spirit was not. She touched people's hearts and inspired everyone she met along the way.

Before we left Boston, I had made appointments for Meaghan to see both her pediatrician and a psychiatrist. Spaulding had provided a psychiatrist, but neither Meaghan nor I felt comfortable with her. She was temporary, and I felt that if Meaghan needed to talk or needed medication, I wanted someone we chose and that Meaghan felt at ease with.

The day of the appointment, Jimmy went with us to help with the car transfer, but his help was not needed as Meaghan and I were now comfortable enough to do the transfer alone. Meaghan met the psychiatrist alone and afterward, with her permission, he discussed his assessment with me. He felt that Meaghan was handling her situation very well. He said that she was emotionally strong, realistic, and not depressed. He also said that she was adjusting incredibly well to her new circumstances. He told Meaghan that if the situation became too difficult for her and she needed help, she should not be afraid to ask for it. He told her that talk therapy and anti-depressant medication may become an option, but for now she was doing remarkably well.

Our next visit was to the pediatrician. We had left his practice when the kids became teenagers and were "too cool" to go to him. I called him from Boston and told him what had happened and asked if Meaghan could return to his practice. There was no one Meaghan or I trusted more, and he would become an ally and advocate for us as we negotiated our new world. After we met with her pediatrician, he also felt that she was doing well considering all she had been through. We told him that she was continuing to have bladder problems, and he placed her on a prophylactic to try to prevent infections. He then called the urologist at Boston Children's, whom he knew personally, to discuss options for Meaghan.

Meaghan mentioned that she had been given a shot to stop her periods prior to chemotherapy and that in her physical condition, periods were the last thing that she needed to deal with. She asked him if he would give her the same shot. She asked him if he would be involved in her case because, unlike other doctors, he listened to her. Meaghan valued his opinion and trusted that he would always tell her the truth. Lesson XV: Trusting your physician and being truthful are crucial to your treatment and success.

Each week, part of our routine was to see the oncologist at CHKD who would oversee the remainder of the study and send the data to Boston. This meant weekly trips to the clinic in Norfolk. Part of the study included an MRI prior to beginning the next round of chemotherapy to see the effects that the radiation and chemotherapy had on the remaining tumors. The MRI was of both the brain and spine, was ordered with and without color contrast, and would take over three hours to do. (Contrast is a dye that is administered during the MRI to help the radiologist determine the separation of the normal and abnormal areas of the brain and spinal cord.)

We were told it would be several days before a report was available so we would have to be patient, which was just another way of saying, "Don't call us; we'll call you." Lesson XVI: Within a short time after an MRI is completed, the radiologist reviews the scan and then dictates the results to a recorder. Radiologists can determine quickly if there is an area of concern, especially if they have previous scans of the patient to compare with. The patient is made to wait so the medical staff can type the report.

Janice Herrity

It was several days before we received the call that there was only one remaining tumor left, at C-7, and it was smaller in size! We were ecstatic by the news; the radiation was successful. Now it was time for the chemotherapy to finish the job!

Meaghan had been on a four-week break from chemotherapy and was to begin her first maintenance dose on August first.

Prior to chemo, she needed to see the oncologist to make sure that her blood counts were high enough to proceed.

Her blood work showed that she was strong enough to handle the chemotherapy, and I was given the okay to give the chemotherapy drugs that night. The Temozolomide dosage had increased, and the drug Lomustine (CCNU) was added for the first day of each cycle. Meaghan's protocol was that she took ten chemo pills the first night and then five pills each night for the next four days. She swallowed the pills with ease, turned on her iPod, put on her headphones, and went to sleep. I must admit that I was very nervous about giving her chemo. I had watched the nurses give it to her each night at Spaulding, but they were nurses - I was not. The first time I gave Meaghan the chemotherapy drugs, I had a friend come over and re-count the pills to make sure that I did not make a mistake. I was so nervous that I stayed up all night to make sure that she had no side effects, which was fine because I still had a good amount of unpacking to do.

Chapter 6 – The Good, The Bad And The Ugly

> *Cancer in childhood occurs regularly, randomly, and spares no ethnic group, socioeconomic class, or geographic region.*

By early August, we were feeling the financial strain of both a medical crisis and the slowing housing market. Our house had been on the market for three months with no offers and little activity, so we decided that the best financial decision was to rent it. Within days of listing the house as a rental, the rental agency received a call from a man who had just put a contract in on another home in the area. He had just returned home to Ohio to show his choice to his family when he saw our listing on the internet. He wanted the house, sight unseen.

He told the real-estate agent that he was a minister and that, "God told him to rent our house instead of the one he had initially chosen" and that he wanted the house in early September. We were so relieved to have a renter and hoped that God had also told him to pay us more than we were asking in rent, but we were not that fortunate. Having a renter in our home was such a relief, and the monthly rent covered all expenses associated with the house. We tried very hard not to show Meaghan that we were under financial stress on top of everything else, but because Meaghan was a teenager, she was acutely aware that her therapy was not entirely covered by insurance and that her illness must be costing us a fortune. We both tried to assure Meaghan that her health was more important than money and that we would gladly sell everything we owned, including our souls, to save her. Although if there is such a contract, I'm certain that the fine print excludes altruistic deeds.

Because Meaghan was considered physically disabled, we were able to apply for Medicaid as a secondary insurance to assist in her medical bills. Even though Medicaid would save us thousands each month in co-pays and would provide Meaghan with a nurse's aide, we felt strange submitting an application as there is a stigma associated with receiving help, especially from the government. We were interviewed and approved and received what is called a Medicaid Waiver. I would have never known that this program existed, but the social worker at Spaulding told me about it. As our journey continued, we would meet many middle class families who were able to pursue and receive the Medicaid Waiver, therefore avoiding financial ruin. Lesson XVII: Call your local social service agency, especially in the case of a child, and discuss your situation. They may be able to assist you.

By the end of August, Meaghan moved back to her bedroom upstairs, and she could enjoy the first independence and privacy since her nightmare began. She had regained many of the neurological losses associated with a spinal cord injury and was walking with a walker more and more. She was beginning to climb stairs and was strong enough to get herself on and off the stair lift without assistance. The effects of the steroids on Meaghan's face were becoming less noticeable, and her level of activity made it safe for her to lose the anti-embolism stockings.

Meaghan was still very uncomfortable with her appearance, as much of the steroid weight remained, and she wore leg braces most of the day to assist in her daily activities. She had lost enough weight that she could once again fit into junior size clothing but was still uncomfortable going out in public, so she turned to online shopping with a vengeance. Although Meaghan was making remarkable strides with her recovery, her emotional scars had not disappeared. Her insecurities had deepened, and she became more reclusive.

Meaghan was certain that her peers were going to reject her because of her appearance, so I think she decided to reject them first. Almost daily her friends would call to see if they could visit her. I would relay the request to Meaghan, and she would usually say that was too tired and that perhaps they could come another day. One day I realized that I could no longer enable her behavior and told Meaghan that I was tired of making excuses for her, that she couldn't hide any longer, and that she needed to reenter the world.

I told her that I understood her fear and that she wouldn't have to do it alone. I would be at her side. I then asked her if she would discard a friend due to a change in physical appearance. She replied, "Absolutely not." I suggested that she needed to consider the moral fiber of her friends. Perhaps her fears were baseless and just teenage angst. After our discussion, Meaghan realized that she couldn't avoid her friend's any longer and turned on her cell phone for the first time in over two months. To her surprise, she saw hundreds of missed texts and calls. That day she started to feel like her old self again and came to the realization that her friend's opinion of her hadn't changed. They wanted to help in any way possible.

Meaghan's Story

Meaghan's fifteenth birthday was a few weeks away, and I was asked by one of her friends what we were planning to do (which was nothing). They asked if they could throw a surprise party for Meaghan. I thanked them for their kindness, gave them our blessing, and told them that we would pay for everything. I told them to invite whomever they wanted, but there was one stipulation: Meaghan tired so easily that the party would have to be in the daytime. Her friends had not had a daytime birthday party since elementary school, but they quickly agreed and took care of all the details.

The night prior to the party, Tropical Storm Ernesto blew into town, and the wind ripped the siding off both houses and left much of York County without power. By noon our power returned, and the party was on. Jim took Meaghan out for ice cream while the girls and I decorated the house. Jimmy and TJ picked up party trays, drinks, and pizza, and by the time Meaghan and Jim returned home, over fifty of her friends had arrived. The idea of a surprise party quickly disappeared as Meaghan and Jim climbed the front stairs and walked into the house past dozens of pairs of flip- flops in a pile near the front door. Her friend's yelled, "Surprise," and many cried as they saw Meaghan walking for the first time.

The party was a success. Not only did her friends come, so did many parents who had not seen us since our days at CHKD. Laughter filled the house, and Meaghan truly felt touched by the outpouring of love and support.

Once September arrived, I needed to address Meaghan's educational status with the high school to have her considered "Homebound" for her sophomore year. Although Meaghan could have benefited from the social aspect of high school, she was not physically strong enough to attend. Furthermore, the numerous medical appointments would only have complicated the situation, so homebound was really the only viable solution.

I was advised that the school district's policy would only provide tutors for a total of ten hours per week and that the tutors were for the basic subjects – Math, English, History, and Science. I was told that much of the instruction would become Meaghan's and my responsibility and that in the past, the high school had had very little success with homebound students, and they had never had a student considered homebound for an entire school year. Meaghan wanted to take seven classes so she could graduate with an advanced degree, so we decided to enroll her for three more online. We figured, "How hard could it be?" Well, it was harder than we both expected. The reading and class pace was a great deal more than Meaghan and I had bargained for, and she withdrew from the online classes within a few weeks.

Janice Herrity

TJ was at the same high school as Meaghan, so he would pick up class assignments daily and return the completed work to her teachers. This was a huge help to me and one less thing on my daily "to do" list. The high school was kind enough to place Meaghan with teachers that the boys had in the past, which made communication easier as I was familiar with each teacher and how they worked. In addition to being quality educators, they were also great people. Each teacher was compassionate about Meaghan's situation and always willing to help if she needed additional clarification or assistance on assignments.

Meaghan's days were hectic. She had occupational and physical therapy three times a week, aqua therapy twice a month, chemotherapy monthly, weekly visits to Norfolk to see the oncologist and, of course, high school work. We quickly learned a new routine. Meaghan would study in the car on the way to therapy and the hospital. I would read the material in advance and create lesson plans and teach as we drove, but I drew the line at math and left a great deal of that to the professionals!

Her tutors would bring the tests from school and administer them, and our routine worked beautifully. The teachers offered accommodations and a shortened workload due to her illness, but Meaghan would not hear of it. She did what the class did. Because Meaghan was not physically on par with her peers, she compensated by becoming an outstanding student and finished the year with an astounding 4.0 GPA.

Meaghan once told me that because she was physically handicapped, she would have to excel mentally to compete in the world. She was no longer a child and looked at her world with a new set of eyes. I was very proud of how she handled both the physical and mental challenges of fighting cancer. She had a maturity and grace well beyond her fifteen years.

Throughout the following months, life began to return to some degree of normalcy for Meaghan. She was able to attend parties again and often needed assistance, so I went to each and every one with her. Sometimes I would get her safely inside and then sit and read a book in the car. Most often I would go inside, find the chaperone, and chat. Meaghan never minded that I came, and if she got tired or needed help, her friends would come find me – it was never an issue. She kept up her social life each day with Facebook, texting, and instant messaging, and her friends came by almost every weekend to watch a movie or just chat. Her fear of rejection was completely unwarranted, and her circle of friends truly helped save her life. Lesson XVIII: It is my belief that when others give up on you, you give up on yourself. Friends are the best medicine of all.

Meaghan's Story

By late fall, Meaghan had progressed so far in her physical recovery that she no longer needed a walker. She was using crutches, which were more "age appropriate," and the wheelchairs we purchased months earlier sat unused in our home. The only wheelchair we used was the one in the car to get around stores or to enter rehab or CHKD, as the pavement and weather conditions were often unpredictable.

Meaghan's back and hand pain had subsided, and she stopped taking morphine on a daily basis. She also regained most of the fine motor skills she had lost and took a break from occupational therapy.

Due the location of the tumor and the surgery, Meaghan had to learn to write again. As an educational accommodation, the school allowed her test answers to be dictated to her tutors. Meaghan had become so strong that by the end of October she was able to take tests without help and write her own essay answers. She also began to walk around our house with only her leg braces and required little to no assistance in most daily activities, even though I continued to be close by should she need support.

Meaghan had another routine MRI at the end of October that showed that the remaining tumor continued to shrink. Everything was positive, and we were all looking to the future for the first time since April. Meaghan wanted a puppy, and we told her that when she was strong enough, she could have one. She was relentless in her pursuit and found the dog she wanted: a four-month old female German Shepherd in Richmond, sixty miles away. Easy enough – nope not for us. By the time we agreed to purchase the dog, the owner was working out of the country, so the remaining puppies had been sent to a breeder in Ohio. In addition to the cost of the puppy, we then had to pay airfare to have the puppy returned to Virginia!

On the nineteenth of November, Molly arrived, and bedlam ensued. Meaghan was thrilled - the other two dogs, not so much. So, for the next few weeks I walked around with a puppy in my arms to stop her from tripping Meaghan and to keep the other dogs from attacking her.

I remember Thanksgiving Day. Meaghan decided that she was strong enough to walk around the house without leg braces or crutches for the first time. She held on to the counters in the kitchen for support. The dogs were fighting, and I was trying to get a turkey out of the oven safely. It was crazy but absolutely wonderful.

I also began to put our own touch on the house. When not driving to therapy, teaching school, or house training the puppy, I began to strip the ugly wallpaper which was everywhere in the house. Stripping wallpaper is a messy job. Meaghan was walking around piles of wet paper, and water was everywhere. So I decided it was best to hire someone and to make sure she was safe. Once the wallpaper was removed, we needed to paint, so we hired someone to do that as well. I now look back at the timeframe and think I must have been crazy to take on such big projects during her recovery. But at the time, it just seemed like the normal thing to do. I think it gave me some control in a world that was out of my control.

One of the side effects of a serious illness in a family is that the other children get pushed aside. Since Meaghan became ill, our focus was on her, her illness, and her treatment. I regretted not being able to help my other children, but that's part of the collateral damage of cancer. TJ was a senior in high school and needed to apply to colleges for the following school year, however we had not given this milestone in his life any real thought or discussion. He had scored 1200 on the SAT and had a good GPA, but we had not toured schools or even discussed what he wanted to major in or where he wanted to go.

I remember telling TJ that since Meaghan's health was so uncertain and his dad traveled during the week, he needed to apply to state schools within an hour or so from home. This was for my convenience, not his. He looked at the options and didn't have the SAT scores for William and Mary, so his decision was easy. Without complaint, he applied to Old Dominion University and was accepted. ODU is minutes from CHKD, so I could stop by on the way to the hospital if he needed anything. It was a very good match for all of us. Jimmy was in his third year at the community college and he, too, needed to figure out where he would go the following fall. He was older, so the restrictions we placed on TJ's search were relaxed for Jimmy. He applied to various schools, but ultimately chose ODU for the same reasons as TJ: to be close to home and near Meaghan.

In early December we went to the orthodontist, and Meaghan had her braces removed. She had worn them for over three years, and she absolutely hated them. She complained every time she was on chemotherapy that the braces made everything she ate taste like metal, and she counted down the days until they were off her teeth. After they were removed Meaghan was elated. She had lost most of the steroid weight, and now, without braces on her teeth, she began to feel good about her appearance once again.

Meaghan had another MRI right before Christmas, and the area looked radically different from previous scans, so the radiologist report was rather vague and inconclusive. One of surgeons that had initially operated on Meaghan felt that the tumor was either dead or that only scar tissue remained. However, the oncologists in Boston and CHKD were not as confident and continued to tell us how difficult GBM was to kill. Jim's research led him to the same conclusion, and he continued

Meaghan's Story

to talk to other brain tumor patients online and developed a strategy if indeed the tumor did regenerate itself. Lesson XIX: Get a second opinion even if the news is good, because cancer has a tendency to "hide." It only takes one mutated cell to regenerate a tumor.

Meaghan's protocol called for her to continue on the chemotherapy for two more rounds, and we were very hopeful that she was going to be the one to beat this. Meaghan had already proven the doctors wrong on several occasions, so we were cautiously optimistic. We had a wonderful Christmas and New Years, and we were all looking forward to a new year with new beginnings. We hoped that 2007 would bring a return to Meaghan's health and that she would soon reclaim the life stolen from her nine months earlier. I would often say to Meaghan that if a miracle came and she was healed, we would never be the same people we were before her illness. In fact we had changed drastically from the people we were prior to her illness. We had all realized that the silly things we often fretted and stressed over were just that – silly. The important things in life are free.

I remember one fall afternoon Meaghan and I sat outside listening to the birds, smelling the freshly cut grass, looking at the blue sky, and admiring the colors of autumn. Had Meaghan not been ill, I'm certain that we would have never taken time to enjoy that moment.

Illness has a way of reshaping your worldview. Some choose to become bitter, but we chose to embrace it. For us, embracing the cancer meant that we were in control, not the disease, and that gave us hope for the future and the strength to fight each day. We had seen and experienced the world of childhood cancer firsthand. If there is a hell on earth it is witnessing innocent children fight this terrible disease.

Yet children accept their situation without question, and oddly there is joy in a pediatric oncology clinic. I met a young woman in Boston who had come to work in this field after her sister lost her battle to cancer several years earlier. She told me that her four-year old sister thought all children went for weekly chemotherapy because all her friends were at the clinic, and they also had cancer. Her sister never feared the disease or the treatments, because she never knew a world without chemotherapy. It was her normal.

I listened as the young woman talked, unable to find the words to express my sorrow that this was her sister's reality. All I could do was sigh. We had witnessed a world that most people do not want to know exists, and I admit that I was one of the many who donated money to St. Jude's, CHKD, and Children's Miracle Network but turned the channel quickly when they interviewed the sick children.

Janice Herrity

In early January, my sister Karen was informed that had she become immune to chemotherapy and that the tumors in her liver were continuing to grow. Her medical options were becoming increasingly limited, and since surgery was not an option for her, she decided to have radioactive microspheres injected into her liver to try to kill the cancer. Karen chose to try the microspheres because they were designed to deliver internal radiation directly to the tumor, since traditional radiation would not have benefited her.

Her treatment was experimental and therefore not covered by insurance. The cost was one hundred fifty thousand dollars. She was very hopeful that this was the answer to her health problems, but unfortunately this treatment would prove to be disastrous for her. There was a medical complication with both her anatomy and her hepatic vein, and the doctor had difficult injecting the microspheres. The treatment did not work, and the microspheres migrated to her stomach where they caused an ulcer, which made Karen vomit almost everything she ate. So in addition to fighting cancer, Karen had another serious health issue that needed immediate attention. Her oncologist placed her on chemotherapy, but with the ulcer she was unable to handle the side effects and had to stop chemotherapy for several months while waiting for her stomach to heal.

The New Year brought a new series of unforeseen challenges. My mother had a series of falls and was beginning to forget things. One afternoon, my sister-in-law stopped by to visit my mother and found her slumped over, slurring her words, and incoherent. She immediately called the paramedics. My mom was rushed to a nearby emergency room, and the doctors concluded that she had a transient ischemic attack (TIA) or a mini-stroke. My mother was admitted to the hospital for a few days and then sent home. Once home her episodes continued and she was readmitted. This time the diagnosis was dementia.

My mother had been a diabetic for many years, and her blood sugar was always under control, but due to the dementia, she had forgotten to take her medicine, which caused her blood sugar to skyrocket. My father was completely overwhelmed by my mother's medical condition and needed help. His solution was to send her to live with either Karen or me. His reasoning was that because we both had ranch homes with extra bedrooms, it would be the ideal situation for her. Although he was keenly aware of both our situations, he was thinking only of himself.

I was totally infuriated with his "solution," and I told him that neither Karen nor I could give mom the care she required and that the best place for her was at home amid familiar surroundings. (I had learned that lesson with Meaghan; The patient is happiest in their own environment.) Even though I would have loved to have my mom live with us, cancer had rearranged our lives, and it was not a realistic solution. Karen and I

Meaghan's Story

both told him that he needed to step up. With the help of my brother and sister, he would do fine. Modern medicine has come a long way in treating dementia and within a few weeks the medications began to work, and my mother began to show signs of improvement.

Meaghan was due for another round of chemo in January, but she could not receive it as her blood work showed that her ANC (absolute neutrophil count) was too low. Neutrophils make up sixty percent of white blood cells, and if there are not enough white cells, chemotherapy cannot be given because chemotherapy kills good cells as well as bad. ANC is how doctors monitor the patient's immune system and gauge how well it is responding to the chemotherapy.

Meaghan would "bottom out" around three weeks after chemo and then her ANC would rebound by the time the next treatment was to be given. The study protocol called for a 1500 ANC level, but hers was less than 800. We tried the next week, and then the following week, and the same scenario continued until Meaghan was finally able to receive chemotherapy a month late. We were very concerned about how the delay would affect her, but the doctors explained that giving chemotherapy to a body that is not strong enough to handle it is far more dangerous than delaying treatment.

I had been in this world long enough to know that there were drugs that could be given to boost her Neutrophils and asked the oncologist about them. He wanted Meaghan to rebound on her own. As I write this two years later, I often wonder what would have happened if I had demanded that Meaghan get the neupogen shot, but knowing what I know about glioblastomias, I sincerely doubt that neupogen would have made a difference.

Meaghan's braces had been off a for little over two months when she began to feel pressure on her front teeth. Her retainer no longer fit comfortably, so we went to the dentist and discovered that her wisdom teeth were coming in, and, of course, all four were impacted. Our dentist consulted with her orthodontist, and they felt that after she had her wisdom teeth removed, she would need braces once again to realign her teeth. (The orthodontist felt so bad about the situation that he told us that this time the braces would be on him.)

We were then referred to an oral surgeon who would do the surgery. It was imperative that we arrange the surgery around Meaghan's chemotherapy schedule and ensure that she was not toxic and that her blood counts were high enough to fight off infection. The oral surgeon was wonderful. He told us that he would do the surgery when Meaghan was strong enough to tolerate it and that we wouldn't need to schedule the surgery until a few days before she was ready. He would work around

Janice Herrity

her schedule. The oral surgeon consulted with the clinic and then had them order a numbing mouthwash for Meaghan's mouth pain because every drug Meaghan took, even over the counter medications, needed to be cleared with the oncologist to avoid any possible drug interaction.

By the beginning of March, I saw ominous signs that things were changing in Meaghan's body for the worse. Meaghan began to tire easily. One day while walking in our house, her left leg began to clonus, which it had not done in months. (Clonus is an involuntary muscle reflex that occurs when the muscles stretch. It is often a sign that there may be something wrong neurologically. It can be identified by a shaking in the muscle.) I immediately panicked and called the physical therapist. He said that the clonus could be due to overuse but strongly suggested that I call the oncologist. When we went to see the oncologist later that week, I told him that things were changing slightly in Meaghan's body, and then Meaghan told him she had begun to feel pain in her neck once again. I almost fainted due to shock because Meaghan had never mentioned the pain to either Jim or me! I was in complete disbelief. When I asked her why she didn't tell her dad or me, she replied that she didn't want to upset us!

The oncologist ordered an MRI to assess the situation, and unlike previous MRI's where I would call to get the results, I did not call for this one. I waited for her appointment the following week because both Meaghan and I knew in our guts that the tumor had regenerated itself. When we met with the oncologist, he confirmed our fears and showed us the scans. There was a white ring around the mass at C7, the same area a few months earlier some had thought to be either a dead tumor or scar tissue from radiation.

The oncologist said that she had just gotten Meaghan's report and would talk to Boston about treatment options. Although I had suspected something was wrong, I felt like I had been sucker punched. Meaghan handled the news better than I did. She was fooling around making jokes, so I would not cry... she hated seeing Jim or me cry. Meaghan used humor as her defense mechanism and had learned to mask her pain with comedy, a trait she learned from the master of avoidance, me.

Once our appointment was over, I called Jim, who was working in Phoenix, and told him the MRI results. He also felt sucker punched but had been researching treatment options in case this scenario occurred. His calmness put me at ease. He told me to drive carefully and that he would email me his research. He then asked to talk to Meaghan, and she talked about everything except her scan.

Afterwards, Meaghan and I did what we always did after an appointment - we stopped at the gift shop and got snacks for the ride

Meaghan's Story

home. Once in the car I asked her if she was scared and she said, "Yes, I knew the tumor was back." Meaghan told me that she was terrified that it would migrate to her brain. She said that she had researched GBM's and her research led her to the conclusion "that they turn your brain to scrambled eggs." Meaghan told me that what she had read about the disease horrified her, and she was aware that she might die. She told me that she wanted to live and would do whatever was necessary to do so. I told her that her dad had options in mind. I would read over the research and then we all, including her, would make a decision. I also told her that I knew that a new chemotherapy would be harder than what she was on, but I said, "Hard - not impossible."

I also told her that this was her body and that she could tell us when enough was enough. We would respect her decision. Meaghan then looked at me and said the words that will forever break my heart: "I have to live, otherwise you won't have a daughter." I looked at her and said, "Regardless of the outcome, we will always have a daughter, and that was the dumbest thing you have ever said!"

She just looked at me and said, "I love you, Mama." Meaghan and I discussed the fact that she may not receive the miracle that we were praying for. She told me that she was okay with whatever the outcome was, but she wanted to live. We drove home, turned on the radio, and sang. Although our world was "rocked," we both had learned that life goes on.

Once home, we did school work, ate dinner, bathed, watched reality TV, Meaghan took her meds, and we fell asleep. I read the mountain of research Jim had sent me and then cried myself to sleep.

Chapter 7 – Here We Go Again

> *2,300 children and teenagers will die each year from cancer.*

We were told of Meaghan's recurrence in late March. Jim had created an arsenal of research in the event that the cancer regenerated itself, and we began to educate ourselves on all of our medical options. Jim concentrated on the adult world and I on the pediatric. We were adamant that we needed to keep Meaghan close to home this time, as there is an intangible benefit to sleeping in your own bed and keeping life as normal as possible while fighting illness. I think it helps the patient, both emotionally and mentally, to be in their own surroundings and feel a sense of control and normalcy in a situation that is completely out of control and completely abnormal. I also felt that Meaghan couldn't emotionally handle another lengthy stay in a hospital setting, but if that was her best chance, then we would do it without hesitation.

We focused our search on drugs that were classified as Phase III. These are drugs that have passed FDA approval and could be given at CHKD. Jim and I were convinced that we needed a drug that had a proven track record with gliomas, and we did not want to enroll Meaghan in a study for a "promising" new drug. We also pursued additional radiation, but we were told that Meaghan had already received the maximum amount of radiation that her body could handle. The risks to current and future health were too great. We had surgeons examine her films to see if they could remove the tumor, but surgery would not become an option. We were also faced with the fact that although Meaghan's tumor was a glioblastomia, it was in her central nervous system. The drugs that we were investigating were used on patients with tumors in their brains and may not be suitable or even work in her case. Finding the correct chemotherapy was our only choice.

That weekend was the Field Hockey Frenzy at Grafton, the same tournament at which Meaghan first felt her neck pain a year before. The event was bittersweet for us. A year had passed, and she was still alive, but she was still fighting cancer. Meaghan was determined to attend the event. Since she was unable to play, she became the team coach.

The night of the tournament, her teammates met her at the gym door and whisked her away to socialize prior to their first game. Meaghan had progressed so far in her physical recovery that I no longer needed to "hover," and she had some semblance of independence. She was no longer using her wheelchair and was walking long distances on crutches. If you didn't know her circumstances, you would have assumed that she had a sports injury, not a serious illness.

The first game the team played, Meaghan sat alongside the girls on the bench, chatting and smiling from ear to ear, but I could see a deep sadness in her eyes. (Jim, on the other hand, thought she was having a great time… a true "Men are from Mars; Women are from Venus" moment.) After the game was finished, Meaghan told her teammates that she was exhausted and was going to go home. She wished them luck with their remaining games and the girls escorted her to our car and said goodbye. Once the last girl left, Meaghan burst into tears. Between her sobs, she screamed with anger and despair over her illness. She was angered by the injustice of her illness, tired of being sick, tired of losing her independence, tired of stares from strangers, tired of leg braces, and tired of fighting so hard only to have lost ground. As parents, we were unable to find the words to console her, so we listened through her tears, as we, too, felt her anger and heartache.

Once we pulled into the driveway I asked Meaghan if she was ready to return to the tournament. She quickly replied, "Yes." Jim was completely confused, but he turned the car around without question. Once we returned to the high school, Meaghan sat frozen in the front seat, afraid to reenter the building. She was considering returning home when suddenly there was a knock on the car window. It was the varsity field hockey coach who was taking a break and sitting outside the gym door and had seen us return. Meaghan rolled down her window, and he could tell that she had been crying. He asked her what the problem was, and she replied, "I miss playing, and everyone will think I'm a baby for leaving. I don't know if I can go back inside." He looked at her and said, "Meaghan, those girls would never think of you as a baby. They think you are the bravest, most courageous person they have ever met." His words propelled Meaghan back inside. For the rest of the night she cheered on her teammates and had a wonderful time.

We continued our research throughout the weekend. Jim talked online with individuals and other families who were dealing with the same disease and all equally desperate for a cure. He was able to get first hand recommendations on the drugs we were researching, the side effects, and, most importantly, if the patient had experienced a recurrence since beginning the drugs.

Our combined research led us to three possible options. We had been in the cancer world for close to a year, so were able to understand the medical terminology and make an informed choice. These were the

Meaghan's Story

most promising therapies available. Oddly, they all made sense to us. Listed below were our top choices straight, from the websites:

AZD2171 – Recentin MASS GENERAL. A new drug that shows promise in treating deadly glioblastomia brain cancers, new research suggests. The drug, an angiogenesis inhibitor called AZD2171 (brand name Recentin), suppresses the growth of blood vessels that feed tumors. Phase II study.

Neuradiab – Duke University Medical Center. Neuradiab was developed at Duke University Medical Center as a proprietary therapy for a particularly aggressive form of brain cancer, glioblastomia multiforme. Phase III multi-center clinical trial of the licensed treatment. Neuradiab has been granted Orphan Drug Status by both the U.S. Food and Drug Administration and the European Medicines Agency.

Avastin – Duke University Hospital. Avastin, a relatively new type of drug that shrinks cancerous tumors by cutting off their blood supply, can slow the growth of the most common and deadly form of brain cancer. The study marks the first time that Avastin has been tested against brain tumors, the researchers said. The drug, whose chemical name is bevacizumab, currently is used to treat lung and colorectal cancers. This is a Phase III drug. The researchers tested the effectiveness of Avastin in conjunction with a standard chemotherapy agent in patients with recurrent cancerous brain tumors called gliomas. They found that the two drugs together halted tumor growth up to twice as long as comparative therapies.

After reading and discussing our choices, we felt that Avastin, an angiogenesis inhibitor, was Meaghan's best hope. It was at Duke University in Durham, NC. We were also keenly aware that GBM's are difficult to kill and almost always come back, so we felt that if we could buy Meaghan time with this drug, something new may be on the horizon that could finish the job. Duke is only three hours from Yorktown, which meant Meaghan could remain at home while receiving treatment. My sister was receiving treatment at Duke, so it seemed like a good overall fit.

The next week I spoke with the oncologist at Dana-Farber. We talked about our three options and what we felt was best for Meaghan. The doctor had a Phase I trial to offer, but I told her that we felt that Duke was where Meaghan should go to receive treatment. She agreed and said that she would call the oncologist at Duke. She knew him both personally and professionally and would discuss Meaghan's case with him. She then asked that she continue to be involved in Meaghan's case through shared information. The oncologist at Duke was on vacation, but his office called us the next day and said that he would take Meaghan on as a patient. We needed only to get insurance approval and have CHKD forward all her scans and history as soon as possible. Our appointment was set for the following week.

Duke was not on our insurance company list as a "Center of Excellence" although they are considered the leading center on brain cancer in the country. At first I assumed that Duke was left off the list because of a clerical error, but after careful research, I learned that the reason Duke was not a "Center of Excellence" was that they did not have a contractual agreement with our insurance company to accept a reduced payment. After learning that a center of excellence was a euphemism, we began to take total control of Meaghan's condition and stopped letting the insurance company direct her treatment. Lesson XX: Insurance companies direct patients to certain hospitals for their benefit and to control their costs. They are businesses and will direct you where it is beneficial for them. If time permits, do your homework and make an informed decision on where you believe the best care and treatment is available. It is also very important to know if the hospital/doctor takes your insurance carrier. If not, you will be considered out of network and will have to pay a larger portion of the bill. Another important detail is to check the yearly out of pocket expense for both individual and family. Once you reach that dollar figure, the insurance company will pay one hundred percent. Always ask what the "Lifetime max" is as well. I also learned through my research that as an adult, Meaghan would become almost uninsurable due to her childhood illness.

Meanwhile, my sister Karen had had yet another setback. Her scans showed that the chemotherapy was not containing her cancer, and Duke stopped her chemotherapy. Her oncologist's only advice was for her to go home and call hospice. Karen told me that she took the news hard. She drove around Duke University until she found Duke Chapel and then went inside and prayed. She told me that she asked God to save both her and Meaghan, but if there was only one miracle to give, let it be for Meaghan as she had already lived a full life. Karen told me that she was going to go to another oncologist and get a second opinion, but she added, "He, too, may have nothing to offer, and if that's the case, I die. The worst case scenario is I'll go to Heaven, and that ain't too shabby either." The next week, on our way to Meaghan's appointment, we passed Duke Chapel, and Karen's words resonated in my brain and tears began to stream down my face. My sister had tried for almost three years to beat her cancer and now the reality was that she would soon die.

Our first appointment was at the Preston Robert Tisch Brain Tumor Center at Duke University Medical Center. The center is one of the largest in the country and deals exclusively with brain and spinal cord tumors in both adults and children. We were surprised by the size of the facility and the number of individuals receiving treatment exclusively for this type of cancer. The registration room was full of patients, many in wheelchairs, and sadly, many were alone. The room was eerily quiet with an air of melancholy about it. I think we had spent so much time in pediatric hospitals that we expected the same level of commotion. The quiet was rather unsettling for us all. Like the previous hospitals, we were assigned a medical-social worker. She talked with the three of us and then with Meaghan alone. The social worker wanted Meghan to speak freely about any fears she might have associated with her disease and her new treatment. We would not meet with the oncologist and his team until much later, so we killed time by doing some retail therapy and walking around the enormous facility. We were all amazed at the size of Duke University Medical Center and still could not believe that it was not presented as an option for Meaghan a year earlier.

We met the oncologist and his team early that afternoon. They were professional, informed, and honest. The doctor felt that the Avastin in conjunction with a conventional chemotherapy Ironitecan would be effective in fighting Meaghan's tumor. However, Meaghan could not begin the treatments until the effects of the Temozolomide and Lomustine had worn off. He examined Meaghan and was quite impressed by her overall physical condition and amazed that she was walking and able to move her body with such ease. He said that she would need to have a port-a-cath installed in her chest wall for delivery of the drugs; otherwise her veins would be destroyed.

The doctor talked to us about the potential side effects of Avastin; the most common was the development of blood clots. He also informed us that we might have a problem with our insurance company as many companies were not approving this therapy because it cost approximately fifty thousand dollars per month. Her protocol would consist of forty-eight treatments over a two-year period. He then told us that Meaghan's wisdom teeth would either have to wait, or we would need to get them out as soon as possible because Avastin is a clotting agent and complications could arise from the blood loss. He also said that in the future, chemotherapy would be administered at CHKD, but for the first few rounds we would need to return to Duke, and all future scans needed to be done at Duke. In the meantime, he would send the roadmap for treatment to CHKD. We were to return to Duke in early May for blood work and scans prior to the first treatment.

On the way home, I called CHKD and told them that Meaghan needed to have a port installed. By the time we reached Virginia, they had a date and time set. Duke was working on getting insurance approval, and thankfully, Meaghan was immediately approved. Meaghan participated fully in all decisions and understood the side effects of the drugs and simply said, "Let's do this as soon as possible, so I can reclaim my life."

Janice Herrity

We were all very hopeful and excited that this new treatment would be the answer to our prayers.

My next call was to the oral surgeon to remove her four impacted wisdom teeth and scheduled the appointment for a week after port placement.

Once we returned home, we were greeted by a new disaster. The floors in the dining room had buckled from a water leak in the laundry room and would need to be replaced. The insurance company brought in huge noisy fans to dry out the area and prevent mold. April was not looking any better than the previous months.

We fixed the floors and continued our lives as they had been prior to the reoccurrence. We had learned that illness is easier to manage with a "normal" daily routine. Meaghan continued her regimen of school and therapy and dealt with the pain by adding morphine to her growing list of drugs. Meaghan's port placement was scheduled for April seventeenth, at 6:30 in the morning – ironically one year to the day after her initial surgery. We met with the surgeon ahead of time. He explained the procedure and told us that port placement is day surgery and is very common. He felt confident that Meaghan should have no problems associated with the surgery. Jim and I were not as comfortable. As parents, any surgery to your child is of great concern, but we signed the consent forms, as we had no other choice, and kept our fears to ourselves.

The day of the surgery Jim was working out of town, so Jimmy came along in case I needed a second set of hands. The surgery went beautifully, and we were back home by early afternoon. However, by four that afternoon, Meaghan began to run a high fever, and her blood pressure dropped to 70/49. I called CHKD and was told to get her back to the hospital, as there was a chance that Meaghan had developed Sepsis, a blood infection that can be fatal. I fought the nurses, thinking they were just being over cautious. Only after checking the internet did I agree that Meaghan needed to be seen. There was one problem – it was rush hour, and the roads were gridlocked. I told Meaghan that we would head to the hospital after rush hour. Until then, I would monitor her vitals because I felt it was safer for her to be home. If a problem arose, I could summon EMT's rather than be stuck on the highway.

Around 6:30, we headed back to Norfolk. Meaghan's fever was now down to 99.5. Although her pressure was still low, it had improved, and I felt comfortable that she would not have a problem. The ER personnel were expecting us and took Meaghan in immediately while I filled out paperwork. In order to see if she had developed Sepsis, the nurses needed to draw blood, which is usually done through the port. They couldn't get hers to work, so they decided to draw blood from

Meaghan's Story

her veins. Each time they tried, her veins blew out, and they could not get a sample. After two hours of this nonsense and some voiced displeasure from me, the ER personnel called a phlebotomist from the VAT team. He was able to get the port working within minutes. The doctors determined that there was an infection and gave Meaghan a large dose of IV antibiotics, which brought her fever down, and her blood pressure returned to normal. Around three in the morning, Meaghan was discharged, and we returned home.

The next few days Meaghan continued to run a low grade fever, and by April 22nd, she had developed another UTI and was having a great deal of back pain while sitting. I called the on call doctor and was told to take her to the ER. An MRI was ordered as Meaghan's pain was unbearable. The scan confirmed our worst fears - the tumor had grown rapidly in less than a month. The tumor that was just a spot at C-7 now encompassed both the cervical and thoracic regions of Meaghan's spinal cord. It ran from C-5 to T-2 and was approximately six centimeters in length. Meaghan was immediately admitted to the oncology floor and placed on steroids to reduce the swelling in her spinal cord.

The oncologists at CHKD and Duke quickly developed a new plan because Meaghan needed the new chemotherapy as soon as possible. Both doctors agreed that Meaghan could not wait until May for her first treatment. After much discussion, they decided that her first treatment would be given at CHKD. Because Avastin was a new Phase III drug, the oncologist at CHKD had never given the drug before but was willing to go ahead with it. Duke sent the roadmap and the two doctors worked together to start the drug early. The biggest obstacle was that she had had surgery less than a week before, and the protocol called for at least a two-week healing period before starting the Avastin.

While we waited for the doctor's plan, Meaghan began to make plans for her own death. She told me that she still held out hope for a miracle, but whatever the outcome, she felt that she had had a wonderful life. She told me how lucky she was that she had two parents that loved her. She said that she knew how to love others, and that was our purpose here on Earth. Her youth minister, along with a nun from our church, came to visit and pray with us. When they asked what else we should pray for I said, "Meaghan's healing." Meaghan quickly corrected me and said, "We should pray for all the children on the floor; they also need a miracle."

Meaghan was very calm and mature. She was no longer a child. Her illness and the subsequent journey had matured her well beyond her years. I was so proud of her inner strength and the beautiful young woman she had grown into. That afternoon Meaghan received the first dose of Avastin and Ironitecan. Thankfully she had no reactions to the chemotherapy, and the oncologists didn't feel that there was a need for us to go to Duke for further treatment. Meaghan was discharged the next day.

The following week at the clinic, one of the nurses talked to me privately and told me that Meaghan was being referred to Edmarc Hospice for Children. Needless to say, it was as if all the air drained from around me. She told me that CHKD was not leaving Meaghan and that she would continue to receive treatment, but with her type of tumor and the associated rate of survival, they felt that it was necessary to include Edmarc at this time. She then asked if I wanted to talk to Jim and Meaghan or if I would prefer that she did. I said I would and waited until we got home later that day to share the information. When I told Meaghan and Jim of the hospice referral, they also were devastated. It was just a month earlier that my sister was told to call hospice, however she began a new chemotherapy and was showing some signs of improvement. So, I began to assume the hospice talk was more common than not. I found out later that I was terribly wrong.

A few days later, Meaghan began experiencing both severe diarrhea and abdominal pain, and I could tell that she had yet another UTI. I called the clinic, and they faxed an order to their satellite office for a urine test and told me to drop a sample off. They had only asked for a urine sample, but my mother's intuition told me to take a stool sample as well. I called our pediatrician instead of CHKD because I knew that they would tell me that the diarrhea was a side effect of the chemotherapy. The pediatrician ordered the test on her stool on my gut feeling alone. He had treated our children for over ten years and knew that my instincts were usually right. Meaghan continued to get worse, and by the weekend we were back in the ER. Once again Meaghan's port did not work. The surgeon that installed the port was in the ER for a consult on another patient. Jim grabbed him and explained our fear that a "lemon" had been installed in our daughter and demanded that he check it out. The port was fine; it was just tricky, which often is the case with patients with breast tissue.

Meaghan was admitted again on May fifth while the doctors figured out what was wrong. They initially thought that Meaghan had developed Clostridium Difficle, (commonly known as C-Diff), which is a "superbug" that is very difficult to kill and can be fatal. C-Diff is caused by long-term use of antibiotics, and cancer patients often come down with the strain because chemotherapy kills the good bacteria in the intestines along with the bad. However, the stool sample I provided three days earlier proved to be key, as Meaghan not only had developed another UTI, which had traveled to her kidneys, she also had E-coli.

Meaghan's Story

(Ironically, my sister was diagnosed with C-Diff less than two months after we had this scare.)

Meaghan was discharged five days later and would receive IV antibiotics through her port for the next few weeks to treat both the UTI and the E-coli. The Edmarc nurses came to our house and taught me how to administer the IV drugs and flush Meaghan's port-a-cath. They explained that they are on call twenty-four/seven, and to call them when a problem arose. Their goal is to keep the kids at home for treatment instead of going into the ER. Although we were not thrilled to have hospice on board, they were absolutely remarkable, and Meaghan quickly developed a relationship of trust with each of the nurses. Edmarc also had a social worker that came with the team, so we now had four social workers, CHKD, Duke, York County, and Edmarc… lucky us! Like most families, we were okay with the medical staff, but the title "social worker" implied talking and sharing feelings, and as a family we were not that evolved.

By the middle of May, Meaghan was once again tiring easily. She continued to have occupational and physical therapy twice a week in addition to chemo bi-weekly and schoolwork. Since school was winding down, and Meaghan had met all her state objectives, I asked the principal if it would be possible to close Meaghan out early, so she could focus entirely on her health. The school principal talked with her teachers and they unanimously closed her out for the year. She only needed to take her SOL's, (state testing), which she did and passed. Meaghan had excelled academically through the adversity and finished her sophomore year with a 4.0 GPA. All who knew her were inspired by her courage, strength, and determination. She became a role model to many of her peers who witnessed her fight her disease with dignity and quiet grace.

The interesting thing about cancer, or any serious illness, is the need to remain normal in the most abnormal of situations. My sister Karen's daughter was getting married in North Carolina in early June, and Meaghan was determined to attend. Karen was resolute in the fact that, as the mother of the bride, she would walk down the aisle and not be in a wheelchair. Both Meaghan and Karen were showing outward signs of their illness, and each was unwavering when an obstacle got in the way of something they wanted or needed to do. Karen planned the wedding with help from friends and went with her daughter to pick out her wedding gown, all while connected to a chemotherapy pump and vomiting constantly.

Meaghan, too, was getting weaker from the effects of the chemotherapy. Her protocol was very demanding. Her body would just rebound from one treatment when it would be time for the next. However, Meaghan was determined to go to the wedding, so we attended.

Janice Herrity

She cherished seeing my parents along with other family members that had come for the nuptials, but she especially loved seeing Karen.

Karen was gaunt and frail, and weighed a little over ninety pounds. It was apparent that she was losing her battle against cancer. The day of the wedding, Karen looked absolutely radiant. She wore a long dress that hid her tiny frame and she smiled from ear to ear. Her goal was to hide the fact that she was so sick, and it worked. My mother told Karen's husband that, "Thankfully, we only needed to worry about one of them now."

Meaghan also looked beautiful, but she was once again self conscious from the side effects of the steroids. She had gained some weight, and her face had once again begun to swell, but she had been in the cancer world long enough to know that the drugs were necessary, so she did not complain. Meaghan was too tired from the trip to attend both the wedding and reception, so we chose the latter, and she had a great time.

The morning after the wedding, Karen came to join us for breakfast at our hotel. Meaghan and I knew that it would be the last time we would see Karen alive. Meaghan and Karen hugged each other silently, knowing that this would most likely be their last meeting here on Earth. Their mutual journey had created a special bond, a bond similar to those that have served in a war. Although I had never left Meaghan's side, I could not feel her pain and get inside her psyche the way someone who has felt the despair of cancer can. As we got in the van to return home, my mother looked at both Meaghan and Karen and then said to me, "It should have been me, I'm an old woman." We were there for a family celebration, however an air of sadness was pervaded.

Chapter 8 – Collateral Damage

> *Diagnoses of brain cancers and other central nervous system tumors rose by more than 25% between 1973 and 1996.*

After the wedding, my parents spent a few days with us before returning home. I had been very careful to "sugarcoat" Meaghan's situation to most of the world, including the boys and both sides of our family. I felt it was necessary for Meaghan's psyche, and I wanted to preserve her dignity above all else. Meaghan was getting weaker and relying on me more and more for assistance with her daily routine. My parents were staying with us and began to see firsthand the staggering effects of Meaghan's illness. The heartbreak and shock was apparent on their faces; words were unnecessary. They also saw firsthand what cancer had done to our family. Meaghan was drained mentally, physically, and emotionally. The boys were quiet and withdrawn, Jim was totally exhausted, and I was in perpetual motion caring for Meaghan.

Although Meaghan was very ill, her illness did not dampen her spirits. She was very happy in spite of her situation and continued to push her body each day. But the cancer and side effects of chemotherapy began interfering with all aspects of her life. By the middle of June, Meaghan was often too tired to complete a physical therapy session, and we began to cancel sessions as leaving the house was becoming dangerous at times.

TJ was graduating from high school, and the morning of graduation was a particularly bad day for Meaghan. She was adamant that we attend the ceremony without her and insisted that she would be fine by herself. She wanted the day to be special for TJ, and she didn't want her physical condition to ruin the day for him. I refused to leave Meaghan by herself and decided to stay home and miss his graduation. I had no intention of leaving her and went to TJ to explain that although this was an important day in his life, I could not leave Meaghan alone. He looked at me and said, "It's not a big deal. It's not like I'm the valedictorian or anything, so there is no need or reason for you to go." He understood that her illness made decisions for all of us; cancer has a way of changing plans on a moment's notice, and we had all learned to be flexible.

Janice Herrity

Jim and Jimmy went to support TJ, and Meaghan and I were there in spirit. After his graduation, we had a small family celebration, and the joke was that we were the lucky ones for not going as Jim, Jimmy, and TJ said that the ceremony was long, hot, and extremely boring!

As the summer progressed, Meaghan grew weaker almost daily. I began to worry about how I would be able to get her in an out of the house once the boys left for school. She was often so weak that transferring to her wheelchair became an issue, especially when stairs were involved. Meaghan, too, became concerned about her safety so we decided that she needed to be moved to a downstairs bedroom.

We replaced the chair lift in the garage with a ramp, so there would be one less wheelchair transfer. I called the insurance company and increased the amount of time that the home health aide was to work, so she could accompany us to medical appointments. I also made arrangements with the York County Fire Department to help me get Meaghan into the house on chemotherapy days. She was often so weak after chemo that getting her safely inside our house was a huge concern.

I discussed Meaghan's exhaustion with her oncologist at CHKD, and he believed that she had developed cancer related fatigue. He said it was fairly uncommon in the pediatric world, but she demonstrated many of the symptoms. I then called the oncologist at Duke to get his opinion. He agreed with CHKD and suggested that we try a drug called Provigil. Although the oncologist at CHKD had never used the drug before, he prescribed it, and it began to work immediately. Meaghan regained her mental stamina, but physically she was still losing ground. I talked with the doctors at CHKD, and we decided that we needed to have Edmarc take Meaghan's blood counts at home and eliminate the weekly trips to Norfolk, as they were becoming too dangerous and exhausting for her. We also chose to switch occupational and physical therapy from the hospital to in-home services. Meaghan reluctantly agreed. She knew that she needed to save her energy for school, which was about to begin.

The chemotherapy caused Meaghan to vomit for several days after treatment. To avoid further medical complications, the oncologist ordered fluids for two days afterward to ensure that Meaghan would not become dehydrated. The clinic ordered IV medication for me to administer through Meaghan's port to help with the nausea. They continually changed medications to stay ahead of the chemo's side effects.

Her protocol called for chemotherapy every other Wednesday. By Sunday evening Meaghan was usually strong enough to get out of bed and eat again. The side effects were absolutely horrendous, but she rarely complained. Only once in all those months did Meaghan ever say

Meaghan's Story

that she thought she couldn't continue chemotherapy. That was after vomiting twenty-two times in one day. The next day she retracted her statement and said that she was under duress and that her statement would not hold up in court... she had learned that from watching hours of "Law & Order" each day.

Another unseen side effect was that Meaghan began to vomit the night before chemotherapy in anticipation of the drugs and their side effects. We learned that this was not uncommon; the nurses told us that the mere thought of chemotherapy could cause nausea. Often children who had completed treatment years earlier would come for their yearly checkup, see the hospital, and immediately vomit. To counteract Meaghan's anxiety, the clinic ordered drugs to calm both her nerves and stomach prior to chemotherapy. Fortunately, they worked. We were told early on in our journey that cancer is a rollercoaster, but we began to feel as though we were blindfolded, and the ride was completely out of control.

By late August, the boys were to leave for school. Jimmy had an apartment and moved himself in gradually; TJ was a freshman and living in a dorm. As the freshman move in day grew closer and closer, I began to stress over the logistics of the move and the fact that I was going to have TJ handle yet another milestone in his life alone.

Jim was unable to attend freshman orientation due to work, and I could not leave Meaghan for two days, so we had a friend from Boston be our "surrogate." Because I had such guilt over missing confirmation and graduation, freshman orientation became a big deal to me, and I would apologize to TJ on a daily basis that we could not be more helpful with his transition to college. TJ insisted that it was no big deal and told me repeatedly that Jimmy could just drop him off with a sleeping bag, clean clothes, and Mountain Dew, and when Jim came home he could bring the rest of the stuff.

Nevertheless, I decided that TJ needed to be like everyone else and have the "big move in day" so I made arrangements for a friend to take him. The morning of the move, my friend strongly suggested that TJ might need me and offered to stay with Meaghan so I could be available if he became emotional. (This seemed quite improbable as TJ is quite Vulcan-like in his emotions, but it was always a possibility.) Meaghan agreed with my friend that I should be there for TJ and promised that she would call Edmarc if a problem arose, so I gave in and took him myself. We did the quickest unpack in history. I made his bed (the only time it was made all year) and returned home – all within a three-hour period. TJ didn't need me nor did he get emotional, but I needed to see that he was going to be okay and was grateful that they both persuaded me to go.

September sixth arrived, and Meaghan turned sixteen. It was a joyous occasion but also bittersweet. She was a year older, still fighting cancer, and still hopeful to reclaim the life that had been stolen from her fifteen months earlier. Sixteen is a milestone birthday. We had planned on a "big celebration" (not the MTV version, but a special party), but Meaghan was just too weak, so we put the plans on hold for when she would be healthy. We ordered a cake, and Meaghan's friends and coaches stopped by to wish her a Happy Birthday. She was truly touched by their gesture, but she wasn't strong enough to leave her bed, so her birthday celebration took place in her bedroom.

Earlier that day, Meaghan had physical therapy, and her physical and motor proficiency, especially walking, was becoming more and more difficult. She tired easily and was having great difficulty with her balance and foot placement. It was obvious that she was losing her physical dexterity. Ironically, Meaghan's sixteenth birthday would be the last time she would walk; the cancer and its far reaching effects took her steps away a second time the next day.

When Meaghan realized that she had lost her ability to walk, she was not distraught at all. She simply looked at me and said, "I did it before; I'll do it again." No tears, no self-pity, no anger, just acceptance and an eerie calm. I often wonder if she sensed the end was coming, because I did. A few weeks earlier I had voiced my concerns to her oncologist and the oncology social worker. Although Meaghan's MRI's showed no disease progression, I had a "gut feeling" that she was not going to beat this thing.

There were many strange things happening with her body. Meaghan would be very cold to the touch, and her temperature would read 94 degrees, and within a short time, she would be hot and have a temperature of 101. This happened so often that it became "normal." I remember calling the clinic the first time it occurred, after a chemotherapy session. I told them what was happening with Meaghan's temperature, and no one had an explanation. Their advice was to watch her closely and that the low temperature was okay, but if the higher temperature reading continued for three consecutive thermometer readings, she needed to be seen as there was a chance of infection.

As I said, the swing in her body temperature became so common that the clinic staff were rarely able to get an accurate reading. They would try numerous times and record the "best one" for their records. The only explanation that made sense was that the tumor was pressing on the nerves that stabilized Meaghan's internal body temperature. In addition, Meaghan's legs began to clonus uncontrollably, and I would have to continually reposition them, basically distracting the nerves and muscles to stop the shaking. Nevertheless, life was rolling forward, and

Meaghan's Story

my thoughts were unimportant. I had learned to "sugarcoat" Meaghan's situation to the outside world. I would do the same to Meaghan. I made a vow to myself that Meaghan would never see my fear or doubt, and we would move forward daily, focusing on our goal of beating the disease and helping her reclaim her life.

Life was very hectic that fall. Meaghan had occupational and physical therapy three times a week, chemo bi-weekly, and was a junior taking six classes. She tried seven but had to drop Latin. (It was hard enough to learn a foreign language on your own, let alone a dead one!)

Meaghan was already very weak. The pace and workload of high school coupled with her medical treatments increased her anxiety, and she was terrified that she would fall behind and not graduate with her class. Because she was so anxious, the doctors ordered the drug Ativan to help her deal with the stress. Her fears were baseless as she excelled in all classes and was able to stay on par with her peers. In fact, the work that was sent home was usually finished within a day or two of receiving it, and more often than not she was ahead in her schoolwork. School and homework made Meaghan feel like a typical teenager and gave her something in common with her friends.

One evening I received a call from Grafton High. The teacher told me that Meaghan had been nominated along with three other girls from her class to be on the Homecoming Court and asked if she was interested in pursuing the nomination. I told the teacher that I was unsure, and I handed Meaghan the phone. I heard her tell the teacher, "Sure," and she hung up. Meaghan looked at me and said, "I hope I don't win, and I pray that this isn't a pity nomination!"

Her fears were baseless as she later learned that her friends had begun a grass roots movement for her nomination because they did not want her to feel that she was forgotten. There was no pity involved, only love.

A week later, her class voted a second time and Meaghan won by a landslide. The school called me and said that they were going to announce the news the next day and would call Meaghan in the morning to tell her the results. I kept the secret, and when they called early the next day, Meaghan was both speechless and honored. But she had a new crisis. She needed a dress, and she was too weak to go shopping. She sent me to the mall with photos of dresses that she saw online. I purchased all six dresses for her to choose from and, of course, she wanted to keep all of them.

Prior to the dance, Meaghan was scheduled to have a routine MRI and another round of chemotherapy. The MRI results indicated that the tumor had not changed, which is not a bad thing. It just meant that the chemotherapy had inhibited the tumor from growing and the Avastin and Ironitecan were working. Her oncologist wanted Meaghan to fully enjoy homecoming and offered to skip a round of chemo or move it to earlier in the week so Meaghan would be recovered by the weekend.

Meaghan decided that she wanted chemo but decided to forgo the Ironitecan and received Avastin alone. By Friday she felt strong enough to attend the pep-rally, but she was extremely nervous about going. Her illness had left her virtually homebound, and she had not seen most of the student body in over a year. Meaghan was terrified of how her classmates would react to her… the cancer had returned, the side effects of the steroids were apparent, and she was in a wheelchair.

We had a friend do Meaghan's makeup, because she was afraid I'd make her look like Tammy Faye Baker, and off we went to Grafton. The moment we pulled up to the high school and she got of the car, Meaghan was surrounded by students. Each student told her the same thing – that they were excited that she was chosen to be on the court, that they marveled at her courage, and that they were very happy to see her.

Once inside the school, we met Meaghan's friends, and they stuck close by her side, sensing her fear and insecurity. I, too, needed to stay close, not for emotional support but for physical assistance, so I also got to attend the pep-rally. I am not known for my love of all things "peppy," and I hate marching bands, but I was tremendously moved by the outpouring of love for Meaghan from both the student body and faculty, so it wasn't as painful as I anticipated.

Along with the presentation of the Homecoming Court, the fall sports teams were called to the center of the gym so they could also be recognized. When the announcement came for Varsity Field Hockey to be acknowledged, her friend and teammate, Taylor, pushed Meaghan to the center of the gym floor to be recognized as a part of the team alongside the other girls. The moment was truly magical, and I saw several teachers and students wiping tears from their eyes as Meaghan's teammates hugged her at center court.

That evening at the football game, Meaghan was to be announced as part of the Homecoming Court, but the logistics to get her safely on the football field seemed impossible, so Meaghan asked a friend to be her stand-in. Her friend received Meaghan's roses and sash in Meaghan's place and brought them by the house the next day.

Homecoming and the preparations involved for a teenage girl are chaotic. Factor in fighting cancer and planning an after party, and "pandemonium" best describes the day. The morning of the Homecoming dance, Meaghan became ill and could not get out of bed, so we cancelled hair and makeup, and she decided to rest until the dance. Prior to the dance, her friends were meeting at a restaurant for dinner, then for photos as a group, and then they were off to the dance, but Meaghan had to cancel those plans and focus all her energy solely on the dance and the after party.

    She washed her hair and decided to wear it down. We had a friend come do her makeup (as you recall, it was determined that I am makeup impaired), and she then dressed for the dance. She looked beautiful, and Jim kept taking her picture, which infuriated her. Meaghan was so angry at Jim that she asked me to drive her to the school and that Jim drive separately. (She wanted him to assist with the transfer and make no other contact once we reached the school.) I was told that I could come inside and wait in a hallway and that I would be summoned if needed.

    Once inside the school, Meaghan was met by one of her friends and whisked away to mingle. I could see from my vantage point in the hallway that Meaghan was surrounded by friends, and she was laughing and having a great time. Once she was out of sight, I left the seclusion of the hallway and went to talk with the varsity field hockey coach and a few of the other teachers who were "lucky enough" to be chaperoning the dance. They told me that each day they heard the students talk about Meaghan, and that they all marveled at her strength and courage. They said that the students had felt helpless since Meaghan first became ill and that nominating her for homecoming court was something they could do for her. I began to tear up, which was strictly forbidden in the rules I had been given earlier. So I returned to my hallway and waited to be beckoned.

    Meaghan was wearing a short black cocktail dress, and her legs were up on the leg rests of her wheelchair. Part of the evening was the presentation of the homecoming court from a staircase overlook with the students below. Meaghan told me afterward that not only was she mortified by her physical appearance but also that the whole student body got a glimpse of her "Hoo-Haw" because of the leg rests. She said, "Having cancer is like a gift that keeps giving and giving."

    I stayed in the hallway until I was summoned and then found Jim, who was waiting in the parking lot, and we took Meaghan home. Our next challenge was to get her comfortable and set up the house for the after party. Once we finished putting out the food, Jim and I were sent to isolation in another part of the house, and her friends were left in charge. After a few hours Meaghan began to tire, so her friends asked the other kids to leave so she could rest. It was a very special night for her, and she was truly touched by the outpouring of love from her peers. I was very proud of her that evening. Although Meaghan was physically handicapped, she did not let the handicap define her.

The next week, Meaghan began to feel an intense pain in her left leg that increased with movement. The physical therapist thought that Meaghan may have injured it during one of the transfers, so she instructed Meaghan to keep the leg raised and rest it. The pain continued, and within a few days Meaghan's leg was twice it's normal size and warm to the touch… a sure sign something was wrong, either an infection or a blood clot.

We went to the CHKD clinic, and the oncologist immediately ordered a PVL (Peripheral Vascular Laboratory), a fancy name for an ultrasound that views the blood flow in the veins and arteries. The test confirmed that Meaghan not only had a blood clot in her leg but also two additional clots in her abdomen. She was immediately admitted to the oncology floor and put on bed rest and blood thinners to stop the clot from breaking loose and entering her lungs (a situation that would cause immediate death.)

The oncologist contacted Duke, and together they decided that the Avastin would need to be stopped for a minimum of three months, but Meaghan would continue to receive the Ironitecan on a bi-weekly basis. Our hope was that the Ironitecan alone would contain the tumor until the clots dissolved and it was safe to begin the Avastin again. The doctors made no promises because they were unsure what scenarios would unfold, as Meaghan was so unique in her disease. The oncologists would now need to improvise – there was no roadmap to follow.

As I mentioned, having a child with cancer is a bi-polar experience and Meaghan, too, straddled the world of hope and the world of reality. The night she was diagnosed with blood clots she told me that if she were to live, her life would not be what she had always dreamed. It would be different because of her physical disability, and that was okay. She told me that she could still live a full life and that she had not given up hope for a miracle and fully expected to walk again. She knew, however, that she would have to depend on wheelchairs and leg braces for the rest of her life. Meaghan said, "I'll most likely have to go to a community college to start while I rebuild my muscles and learn to walk again."

She had come to the realization that her dream of being a nurse would never happen because the job would be too physically demanding for her. She then said, "I think I will be a Child-Life Specialist and empower other children suffering from childhood cancer." Meaghan said that she expected one day to get married and knew that she was most likely sterile due to the radiation and chemotherapy and hoped that one day, one of the boys wives would be a surrogate for her. The last year and a half had taught her valuable lessons and had reshaped her vision of the world. I listened as she talked, heartbroken that her childhood dreams had been stolen by cancer.

Meaghan's Story

While waiting for an answer to her latest health predicament, Meaghan and I began to discuss in depth what would happen if the tumor did regenerate and what her options would be. I assured her that her dad and I would continue to look into other therapies, but most were experimental. She said that she had also researched the disease and had come to the same conclusions. Meaghan knew that the clots were the worst-case scenario and said, "I'm hoping for a cure, but I'm going to prepare for the probable."

Meaghan began to quietly make plans for the "probable." She began scrap booking with a vengeance and created three books for us, two of our family and one of her life. Jim and I hated to see her make the books because we knew her motivation, but we reluctantly agreed to buy her the needed supplies. She made numerous Christmas decorations and created a surprise playlist on my iPod of my favorite songs and titled it "For Mom!" Although I hated seeing her prepare us for life after she was gone, I treasure each gift that she created.

Although Meaghan was preparing for the end, she continued to live. She continued to laugh, and she continued with school. She asked that I create a Caringbridge website for her, as she was now ready to share her journey with others.

Chapter 9 – Death & Rebirth

> *Diagnoses of leukemia, which is the most common childhood cancer, increased by more than 15% over the past 20 years.*

Meaghan was placed on the anticoagulant Lovenox to break up the blood clots. Once the doctors determined the correct dosage and prior to her discharge, the nursing staff taught me how to administer the drug. I would need to inject Meaghan every twelve hours to ensure that a steady dosage of the drug was in her bloodstream at all times. Since the syringes were pre-filled, I had to shoot out the excess medication and then rotate areas on her stomach because one of the side effects of the shots was bruising. After a week on the drug, Meaghan's stomach was a canvas of black, blue, yellow, and purple. Each time I gave her a shot, my heart broke, as I knew that within a few hours she would have yet another bruise.

Meaghan was now on over twenty medications. Many were to be given every four hours, so I would sleep about three hours a night to keep the medications in her system at all times. I would wake Meaghan from her sleep at least twice during the night, She would open her mouth, I would drop the pills in, and she would then take a sip of water and fall back to sleep. I became so efficient in my routine that I would lay her medications out in a medicine cup, fill the needed syringes, and label each one prior to bed to save time. Jim created a daily medicine sheet for me, and I would check off the medications that had been given, and their respective dosages, to ensure that no mistakes were made. He and the boys would pitch in when they were home, so I could get some rest. Our system worked quite well.

Our days were hectic that fall. I woke up each morning by six and gave Meaghan her morning medications. I would then give her a Lovenox shot at seven, help her shower, and give her more meds with breakfast. Then there was physical and occupational therapy (twice a week) followed by school, lunch, meds, nap, school, meds, school, dinner, evening shot, homework, meds, TV, email, phone calls to friends,

Janice Herrity

medication before bed, meds at midnight, and meds at three. Because of the blood clots, Meaghan had to go to Norfolk each week for a PVL, and she had to go biweekly for chemotherapy. I credit the power of the human spirit for getting us through each day. Meaghan and I were on a mission, and we would do whatever was needed to accomplish our goal.

One afternoon while Meaghan was getting chemotherapy, we watched the movie *Apollo XIII* and began to draw comparisons between the astronauts' predicament and the complicities of fighting cancer. Meaghan's situation paralleled the astronauts' predicament as she needed to adapt to an ever-changing situation, remain positive, and trust the experts to solve whatever was the problem at hand. Meaghan would paraphrase Jim Lovell and say, "Janice, we have a problem" whenever a new side effect developed (which was often). I emotionally connected to the character that Ed Harris portrayed in the movie and the words, "Failure is not an option." It became my mantra of sorts.

The clinic at CHKD and Edmarc were similar to mission control. They were always a phone call away and would be able to talk me through many situations and helped to keep Meaghan at home and avoid a trip to the ER. When Meaghan's health began to worsen and the outlook would seem grim, I would often say to her, "What's good with the aircraft?" basically saying that although her body was failing, she still had her mind, her spirit, and her personality intact. It was imperative that we both focused on the positive aspects of her situation to get though the predicament.

By mid-November, Meaghan began to regain her strength and looked fantastic. She had seen photos at the clinic taken by Flashes of Hope and wanted to have our family photo taken to include with our Christmas cards. (Flashes of Hope is an organization that takes photos of children with cancer and other life threatening diseases, at no expense to the family.)

Meaghan wanted to keep the photos casual, so she asked that we coordinate our looks. She thought that the photo would look lovely if she and I wore sweaters and Jim and the boys wore collared dress shirts. Her plan seemed foolproof, but the morning of the photo shoot, we met the boys at CHKD, and to our disbelief, they had messed up Meaghan's vision! TJ was in an Old Dominion sweatshirt. When Meaghan asked him if he had gotten the message on what to wear he replied, "Yeah, Mom said a college shirt." Jimmy did have on a dress shirt, but he pulled it out of the dirty laundry. His shirt was wrinkled everywhere, it smelled of smoke and cheap cologne, and to add insult to injury, he had not shaved or showered… because he had just rolled out of bed!

Meaghan's Story

It was too late to send them back to campus, so we cleaned the boys up the best we could and had our family photo taken. To our amazement, the photographs came out beautifully, and we absolutely treasure them.

After the photos were taken, we headed to the mall to shop. Meaghan had lost nearly forty pounds since August and was in need of new clothing. We planned to head to Virginia Beach after shopping to cheer on her field hockey team as they had advanced to the state semi-finals, but by the time we finished shopping, Meaghan was too tired to go, so we came home.

We had a great day, and Meaghan was really beginning to regain her strength. We were so happy and hopeful that maybe our prayers had been answered and she was beating the cancer. Our joy was short lived. The next morning Meaghan woke up with a fever and had developed another kidney infection. She was in so much pain that we could not go to the championship game. This broke her heart. Sadly, her team lost by one goal in overtime. I remember asking Meaghan if it upset her that the team did so well this year without her. Meaghan replied that she was not resentful at all. The girls had supported her through her illness, and she was extremely happy and proud of their accomplishments.

One of her teammates told me later that the loss hurt, but after watching Meaghan battle cancer, she realized it was just a game. This was the first time I began to grasp the impact that Meaghan's illness had had on her peers. Her struggle and the grace with which she handled her situation had a profound effect on these young people's lives. Having a friend with cancer had taught them valuable life lessons about priorities, compassion, and friendship.

The month of November brought much sadness for Meaghan as she knew several children who would die by Thanksgiving. The first child was an amazing eight-year old girl named Nina whom we had met at CHKD while waiting for tests. Nina was diagnosed with cancer about six months prior to Meaghan. Nina was very smart, very funny, and incredibly brave. Meaghan marveled at Nina's tenacity and courage, but after two years of fighting this awful disease, Nina lost her battle.

Meaghan was greatly affected by Nina's passing. Nina was the first child that Meaghan knew personally to die of cancer. Meaghan had a hard time understanding the senselessness and the injustice of Nina's death. Her heart broke for the little girl's family, especially her mother. Meaghan began to feel guilty that she was alive and this little girl had died, and she was very concerned that the little girl's mother would hate her if she received a miracle while Nina had not. I had no answers for her, and I understood her angst. I told her that if she beat this monster, the

Janice Herrity

little girl's mom would be the first to cheer, because there is no jealousy among parents whose children are critically ill.

The next day we received word that a teenage boy we knew from the clinic had lost his battle with cancer as well. The following week, while Meaghan was receiving chemo, a six-year-old boy died in the clinic after receiving his treatment. We were in the treatment room next to the boy, and only a thin curtain separated us. When the little boy began having problems, a code was called, and suddenly there were medical personnel everywhere. I realized what was happening, turned off the movie we were watching, and had Meaghan put in her ear buds and listen to her iPod. Although Meaghan was distracted, she knew that the situation was dire and figured out that the little boy had died. Three children that we knew had lost their battles within one week. This shook Meaghan and me to our cores.

Meaghan was acutely aware of her own circumstances, so when she was assigned to read *Thanatopsis* (a meditation on death) by William Cullen Bryant and then write her own poem on death, I became very concerned that the assignment was too close to Meaghan's own situation and that she wouldn't be able to handle the assignment emotionally. I discussed my concerns with Meaghan and told her that I was certain her English teacher would understand and perhaps assign her another poem. Meaghan insisted that she did not want a different poem or any special treatment because she was sick.

She began the assignment, and within a few hours she had constructed her own poem, which was very insightful and, I believe, cathartic. Meaghan rarely discussed her illness with anyone other than medical personnel and our immediate family. Her teacher was so moved by the poem that she submitted it to a high school publication. It was accepted and published. Meaghan titled her poem Rebirth. The poem is a testament to both her spirit and her faith.

Prior to becoming ill, Meaghan had always written poetry as a creative outlet, but she stopped once she became ill. Because her new world was so scheduled, there was little time to sit and reflect. Ironically, an assignment on death gave Meaghan the needed artistic vehicle to express her emotions and fuel her passion once again.

Rebirth
Meaghan Colleen Herrity

My eyes grow old at the changing colors
Bright orange, crimson reds, golden yellows

Meaghan's Story

Autumn's chilly grasp takes hold of the days
Bitter winds blow from the north, east and west.

The clear blue sky turns to a dreary grey
Trees ablaze with color become barren
The ground is cold and hard beneath my feet
It is covered by a mountain of leaves.

Soon winter will descend upon the Earth
The fresh snow covers the death of Autumn
Beneath the soil, nature is at slumber
The warmth of the sun brings hope for new life.

The empty limbs of trees are green and lush
Their beauty breathes new life into my soul
The aroma of spring wakes my senses
Nature's renewal, behold its splendor.

Beautiful colors lift my weak spirit
I look to the heavens, my soul renewed
The promise of rebirth is now fulfilled.

The week of Thanksgiving, I received some news that shook my world. My sister called to tell me that her cancer had migrated to her brain. It was the worst-case scenario and her greatest fear. Her oncologist immediately stopped chemotherapy and within the week, Karen would be starting radiation. In the three and a half years of fighting this disease, Karen had never had radiation and had no idea what to expect. She called to ask me questions and advice about treatment options. Our roles had now reversed; she was no longer the expert.

Meaghan took the phone and explained to Karen in great detail what she needed to know, what to ask the doctors, what to wear, and even the smell of the ions splitting in the air as the beams of radiation cut through it. Karen was to begin steroids to reduce the swelling in the brain, and Meaghan counseled her on this as well. The conversation was mature and matter of fact. It was a surreal moment, my teenage daughter advising an adult about brain cancer and the subsequent treatment options including their side effects. It literally made me sick.

Later that week the boys came home for Thanksgiving, and we had a wonderful day. We sat in the backyard, played with the dogs, and talked while the turkey cooked. After dinner, Meaghan wanted to get the house ready for Christmas, so we decorated the outside to fulfill her wish. Once nightfall came, we plugged in the lights, and as in years past, the lights immediately blew out. The next day while Jim, Meaghan, and the boys tried to fix the outside lights, I decorated the inside of the house and trimmed the tree.

Our tree is full of ornaments that my children made from preschool through elementary school. Each ornament has a memory or a story; many are from family vacations, Jim's business travels, a past Christmas, or a gift from a friend or neighbor. I also had purchased ornaments for each of our children every year, so that one day they could hang them on their own family tree. By the time I finished decorating the tree, I was in tears. I knew that there was a real possibility that by next Christmas, Meaghan would not be with us, and she would never have her own tree or her own family. The pain was more than I could bear. I blamed my red eyes on the dust from the boxes and carried on, but I was not alone in my fear. We were all thinking the same thing...

Karen began her radiation the following week. The cancer and years of treatment had left her body exceptionally weak. She weighed less than eighty-five pounds. The cancer had returned to her breast and had metastasized to her liver, lungs, and brain. Because she was so frail, she did not tolerate the radiation well. After a few treatments, the doctors and Karen both decided that she was too weak to continue, and radiation was suspended.

Karen had fought this monster for three and a half years, tried numerous chemotherapies, radioactive microspheres and radiation, and still she could not defeat the cancer. She was still full of hope for a miracle; but in case the miracle that she hoped and prayed for did not come, she made plans for her death. Karen wrote her will, gave her husband a list of books to give their unborn grandchild for the next eighteen years, and planned her funeral. Karen was a very spiritual person. She had a degree in theology and read the Bible daily. Like Meaghan, she never questioned why this was happening to her. She accepted her situation with grace and never wavered in her faith.

The same week Karen stopped treatment, Meaghan had a routine MRI and another PVL for the clots in her stomach and legs. The morning of December thirteenth, CHKD called to inform me of Meaghan's tests results. The MRI results came back better than expected - the tumor was a bit smaller and so were the clots. Meaghan was beginning to lift her legs and move her toes again, and the pain in her hands was once again subsiding. When I received the call, we were having new leg braces made and were making appointments for Meaghan's return to outpatient physical and occupational in January. We were both overjoyed by the news. Meaghan looked fantastic and felt great. The wheelchair was the only clue to the outside world that she was ill. However, our happiness was short lived. My nephew called that same evening to say that Karen

Meaghan's Story

had passed away surrounded by her husband and children. They wanted us to know that due to Meaghan's illness they did not expect us to attend her service. Meaghan insisted that we attend. She wanted to say goodbye to Karen. They shared a special bond - one only known to those who fight this terrible disease.

The night before we left for Karen's service, Meaghan received a call from one of her friends. She was having a Christmas party and wanted to know if Meaghan was up to coming. Meaghan told her that she was feeling great, but getting into the house would be a challenge. Her friend told her to come. She said that the guys would lift her inside. She agreed, and off we went to another high school party. By the time we arrived, her friends had moved the party outside and built a fire. They met us at the car and whisked Meaghan away to join them. She had a great time and partied until one in the morning. The next day we got up early and drove to North Carolina for Karen's funeral.

Meaghan attended Karen's wake but was too tired for the funeral service. I was planning on going back to the hotel with her, but Meaghan insisted that I stay for the service. She knew it was important to me and said she would be just fine with Jim. Meaghan never ceased to amaze me with how she always put others' feelings above her own situation. I was so proud of her, and I continually marveled at the young woman she had become. My sister's service mirrored her life. It was a humble commemoration of the three F's (Family, Friends, and Faith). My heart broke for her husband and children, especially my niece, Abby, who was expecting her first child. It was hard to believe that less than six months prior, we were at this very same church celebrating her wedding.

I tried to focus on the service, but my mind continued to wander to thoughts of Meaghan and her illness. In less than one month, we had known four people who passed away from cancer, and three of them were children. I knew I needed to keep my thoughts private and had learned to relish each moment – not only with my daughter but with everyone who was important in my life, as tomorrow is an uncertainty for all.

The next day we returned home and prepared for Christmas, which was less than a week away. Meaghan loved Christmas and had shopped for months to make it special for our entire family. Each day leading up to Christmas we would sit in the family room, admire the tree, sip hot chocolate, and listen to Christmas music.

On Christmas morning, we received a surprise visit from the York County Fire Department. They brought Meaghan a gift and wanted to let her know that they were thinking of her. The firemen had become quite fond of Meaghan and were always so kind when they helped her on chemotherapy days. She was truly touched by their thoughtfulness.

Janice Herrity

Our Christmas was lovely, if quiet and sad. We all sensed that this would be our last Christmas with Meaghan, and she knew it as well. Life was changing quickly for her, and the strength she had regained weeks earlier was quickly disappearing.

Meaghan's physical condition was rapidly deteriorating, and she was in need of special physical therapy equipment because of the time she spent in bed. We needed to purchase a piece of equipment called a stander to make sure Meaghan's bones would be able to support her when she began to walk once again. New standers cost around six thousand dollars, but we could get a used one for two thousand. Jim and I were prepared to pay for it out of pocket as it was a necessity, but I had read our insurance policy and knew that it should be a covered expense if we obtained preauthorization. I tried for weeks to reach someone who had the authority to pre-approve the stander.

After several failed attempts, Jim contacted his personnel manager to see if she could help us. She provided us with a different number than was on the back of our insurance card, and I reached a woman who was authorized to approve the stander. During our conversation, she alluded to the fact that it should be our responsibility to pay for the expense as the insurance company had paid an enormous sum on Meaghan's care thus far. I replied in my sweetest voice that the insurance company is in the business of risk and that they took a gamble and lost. After a period of silence, she agreed to approve the claim, and we were able to get the stander. I then told her that Meaghan needed a custom wheelchair, and as I had her on the phone, asked her to pre-authorize the wheelchair for the following year's medical expenses. She was not amused, but she agreed.

Medical insurance is crucial when fighting illness and can give the patient and family much needed peace of mind. Our primary insurance company was beginning to reject many of Meaghan's claims for no apparent reason other than (and this is purely speculation) that they were tired of paying. I truly believe that the insurance companies count on the fact that people are too exhausted from the nonsense of the medical world to fight a rejected claim and hope the patient will just pay the bill to avoid one more battle. I was tired, but I still had a great deal of fight left in me, so I would call to rectify each rejected claim. There was a myriad of reasons for rejection, ranging from coding errors and non-covered items to exceeding plan limits, etcetera. My favorite "rejected claim" was that I had not answered an informative letter asking if Meaghan was a full-time college student. I explained with great sarcasm, lost on the nitwit that I was dealing with, that like most sixteen year olds fighting cancer, of course Meaghan was a fulltime college student, and she was studying astrophysics at both Harvard and MIT. The representative thanked me for the information and then asked what MIT stood for and where it was located. Not wanting to mess up any additional claims, I explained that it was an attempt at humor. The representative was not amused, and I was then transferred to his supervisor.

By mid-January, Meaghan was again feeling poorly and began to experience painful headaches. She was having difficulty reading and needed glasses to watch television. She began to have seizures and her lower body would clonus uncontrollably. In addition, the intense neck and back pain returned. One morning after bathing, Meaghan had a violent seizure, and her body shook so uncontrollably that she fell out of her wheelchair. I was alone. Our home health aide was out sick, and the boys had returned to school. I tried unsuccessfully to pick Meaghan up, but she was so weak that she couldn't assist me, so I had to call 911. The EMT's arrived and decided to transport Meaghan to the CHKD emergency room to be examined to ensure that she had not broken any bones.

I told her that I would drive to CHKD separately and meet her there. I then called Jimmy and asked him to skip a class (to which he was very agreeable) and wait with Meaghan until I arrived. The ambulance left, and I followed in my car, only to break down at the end of the street. I came home and took another vehicle only to discover that the gas gauge was below empty. While in transit, the instrument panel began blinking and bells began ringing, but thankfully, I made it to the hospital without breaking down a second time.

When I reached the ER, Jimmy was sitting with Meaghan and was in shock from what he was witnessing. Meaghan had regressed so quickly in her physical state that she was almost helpless. I had sugar coated her situation to the boys so they could move forward with their lives, but I could not spin what he was witnessing. He was fighting back tears, and there was nothing I could say, so I threw him the keys and told him to put gas in the car. As I mentioned before, there is a collateral damage with cancer, and I only had the energy to help Meaghan's psyche. I would deal with Jimmy's anguish another day.

The oncologist ordered an X-ray to make sure that Meaghan had not broken any bones. He then asked if I wanted an MRI but warned me that Meaghan had been living on "borrowed time" and that if the MRI showed disease progression, he would stop chemotherapy immediately. His words resonated with me as I suspected that the tumor had regenerated, so I declined the MRI.

I had not been completely forthcoming with the doctor about the changes I had seen in Meaghan's body. I only told him that things were getting worse. I was afraid that if I shared everything, especially the blurred vision, which I knew meant that the tumor had grown and was now pressing on the ocular nerve, he would order the MRI of the spine and stop treatment.

I was fairly sure that the cancer had spread into the spinal cord but not to Meaghan's brain. She wasn't showing any signs of confusion, and her memory and mental function were sharper than mine. I agreed to a brain MRI, but not a spine MRI. Although I was cognitively aware that the chemotherapy had not stopped the cancer, I was afraid that if I articulated those words, Meaghan would lose any chance of restarting the Avastin. In essence, I would be giving her a death sentence because I knew there were no other viable treatment options available for her.

Jim researched GBM's day and night in case Meaghan had another recurrence. The only options were dangerous to her health and experimental. We couldn't do the brain scan that day, so we rescheduled it for a few days later. Thankfully her brain was free of disease.

The following week, Meaghan was scheduled for both chemotherapy and a PVL. The PVL was scheduled first and the results were encouraging. The blood clots still remained, but the blood flow was increasing in both her left leg and abdomen. It was positive news, and we were hopeful that she would be able to restart the Avastin by the end of February – if Duke felt it was safe.

Afterward, we went to the oncology clinic for Meaghan to receive chemotherapy. Meaghan was extremely weak and did not have the upper body strength to assist in her transfers. The decline in Meaghan's health was apparent, and I began to tell the doctor and nurses what I was witnessing each day. I also told them that getting her to the hospital for chemotherapy was becoming too dangerous.

The oncologist discussed having Edmarc administer the chemo at home for her safety, and then he ordered both oxygen and suction for home use to ensure that we had the necessary medical equipment in the event that Meaghan had a grand mal seizure. After the oncologist finished examining Meaghan, and as one of the nurses was administering her chemotherapy, Meaghan began to simultaneously clonus and seizure.

The nurse summoned both another nurse and the oncologist. They all stood there stunned. I was calm. The doctor looked at me and said, "Is this new?" I replied, "No." He then asked me what I did when this happened. I told him that I gave her 1 mg of Ativan through her port. He wrote the order and within a few minutes the episode stopped.

Meaghan was in no pain, and she showed the oncologist that she could pull her legs up. He just looked at her with disbelief. Meaghan was so unique in her disease that her body changed almost daily and, thankfully, the oncologist listened to both Meaghan and me and would adjust her treatment and medication often on our observations alone. I remember him telling me that I was now the expert on this disease because her body reacted like nothing he had ever seen before.

    Each day brought both new challenges and new surprises. One day Meaghan would be able to lift her legs and wiggle her toes, and other days she had no feeling below her abdomen. Her hands would begin to regain dexterity and her pain would subside, but the next day she would have limited fine motor skills and need morphine to deal with the pain. Meaghan was adamant that only the medical world would be aware of her physical changes and she too began to "sugar coat" her situation to the outside world.

    Although Meaghan was slipping physically, she continued to push herself mentally. She had six midterms to take and was having seizures constantly. Her teachers were keenly aware of her health and offered to postpone the exams until she was stronger, but she insisted on taking the tests. In the middle of her American History exam, Meaghan had a mild seizure, stopped the exam for a few minutes, then regained her momentum and continued on. She did not waver; her goal was straight A's for the semester, and she came close – five A's and one B, which was amazing as ill as she was. Her success was a testament to her spirit, and she inspired both her classmates and peers with her positive attitude and commitment.

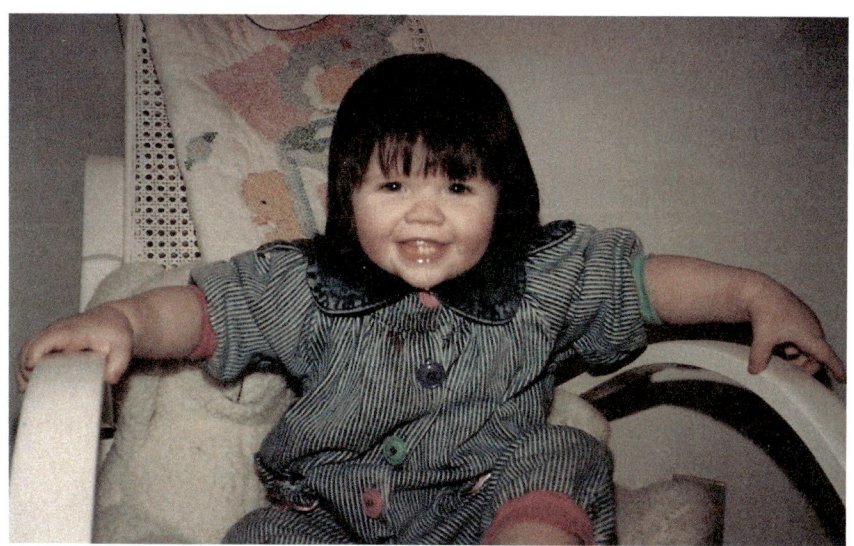

ABOVE: Meaghan at 18 months old – she was always smiling.

RIGHT: Meaghan at two years old playing in her room in New York

BELOW: TJ, Meaghan, and Jimmy in 1992

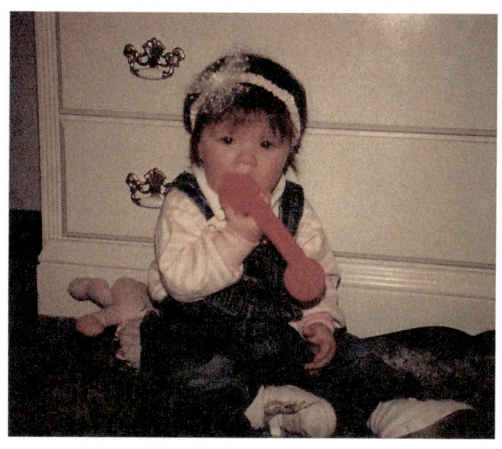

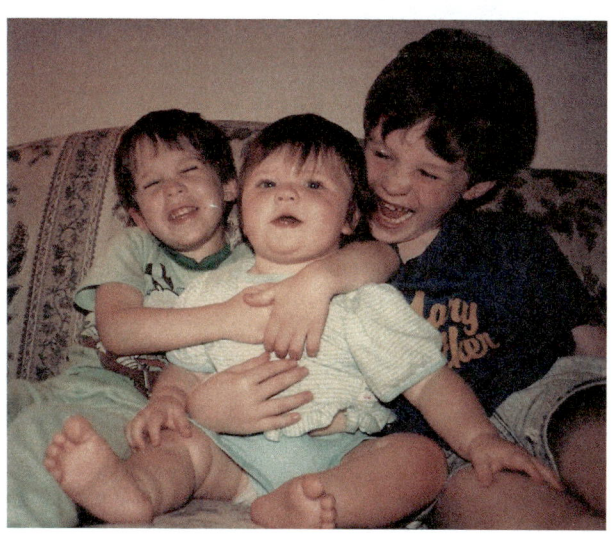

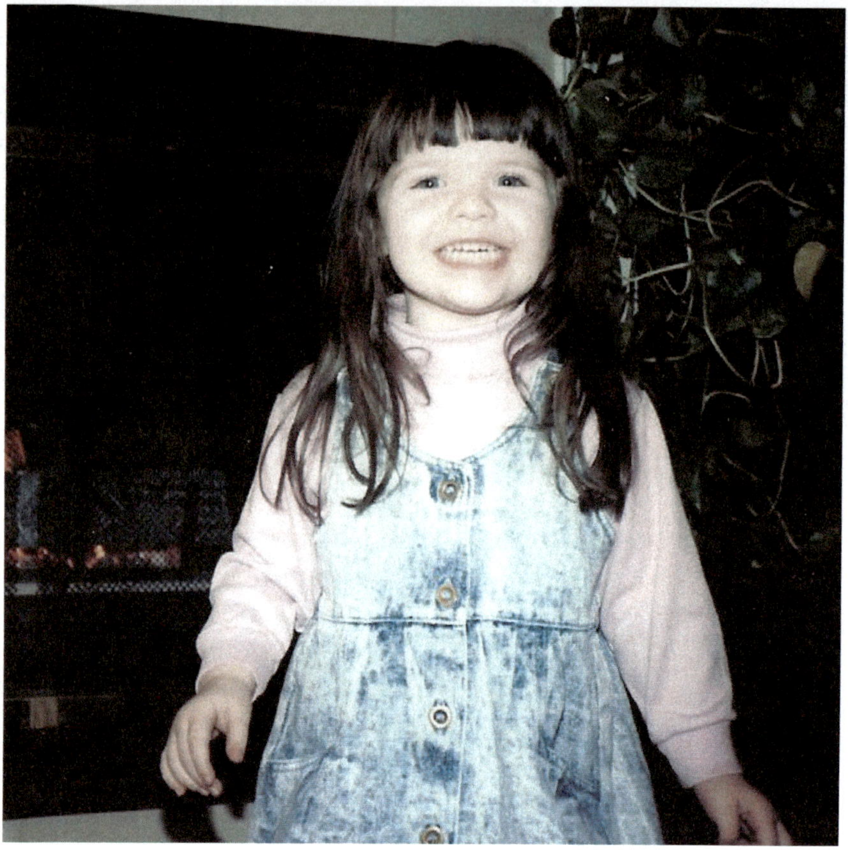

Meaghan, Autumn of 1994

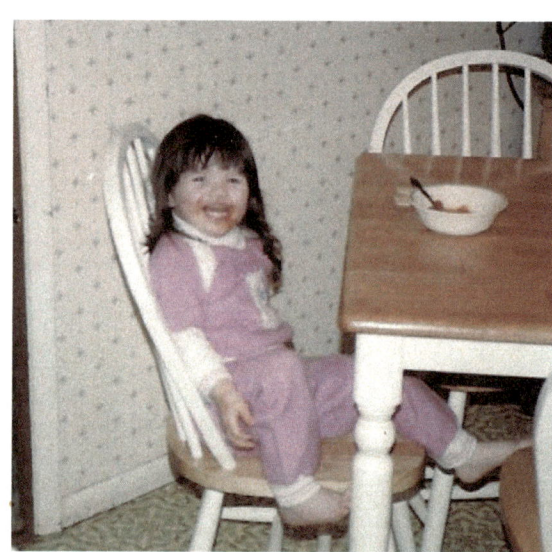

Meaghan eating lunch - there was more food on her face than there was inside of her!

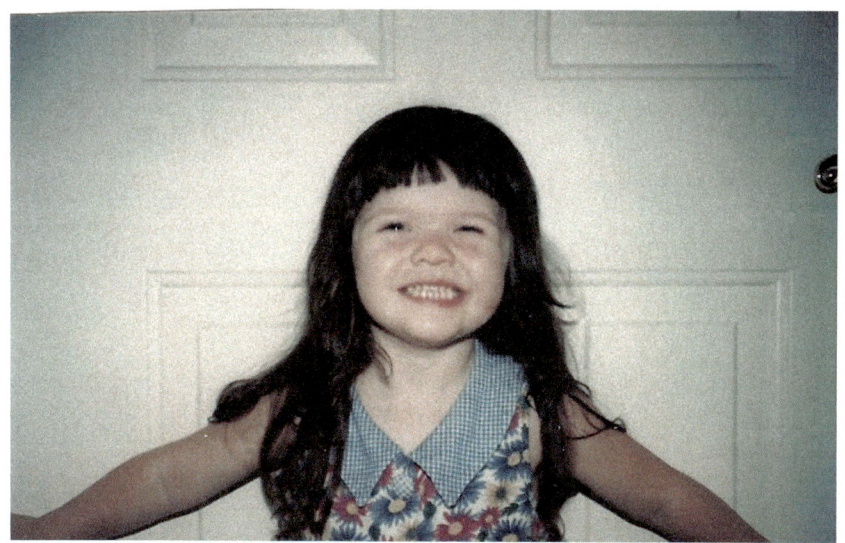

ABOVE: Summer of 1994 - we had just moved to Virginia

RIGHT: Meaghan sunning herself by the pool in St. Thomas, Virgin Islands in 1999

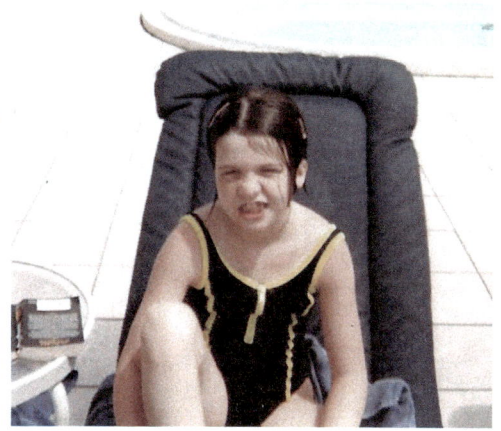

Halloween 2000 - Meaghan was a flower child.

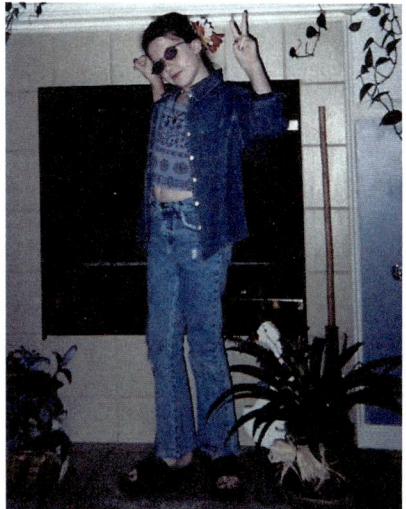

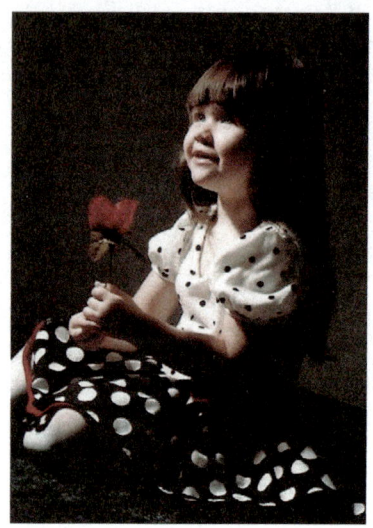 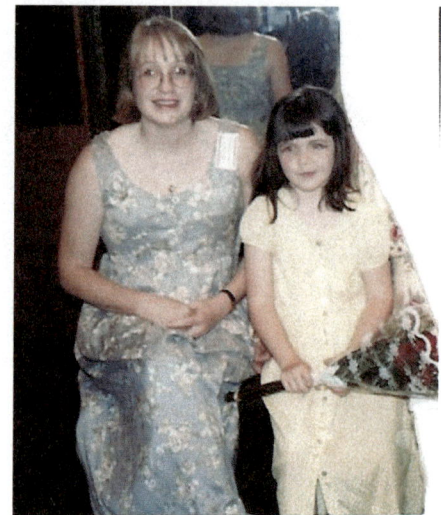

ABOVE LEFT: Meaghan's fourth birthday photo

ABOVE RIGHT: Meaghan and her mom after a dance recital in the Spring of 1997

BELOW: Easter morning of 1995

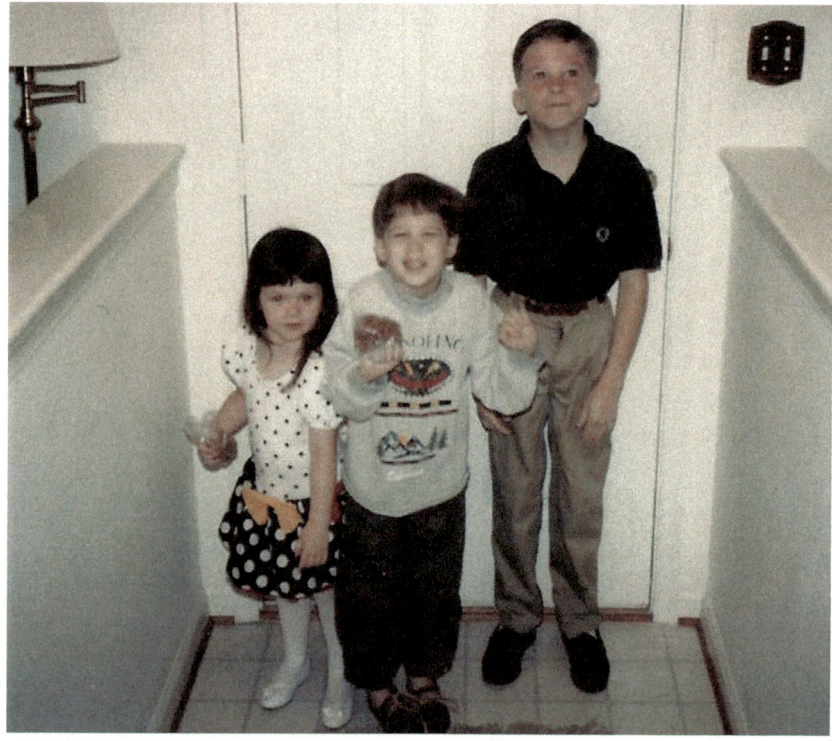

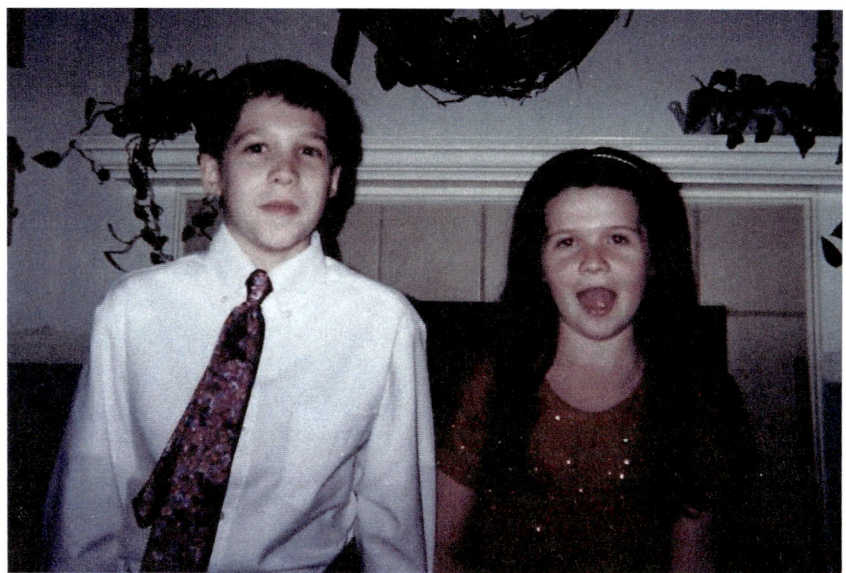

ABOVE: TJ and Meaghan before a school Christmas concert in 1998

RIGHT: Meaghan in her gymnastics phase... she broke three toes later that day when she failed to stick a landing.

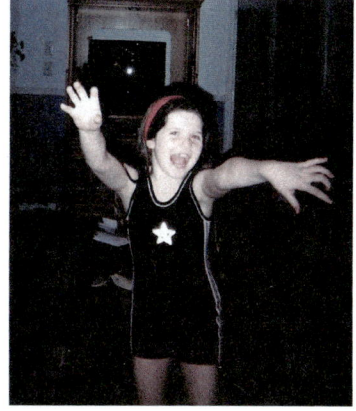

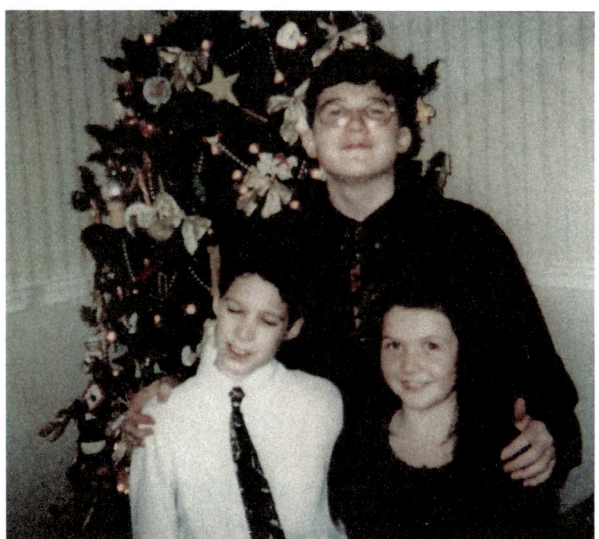

LEFT: Christmas Eve 1999

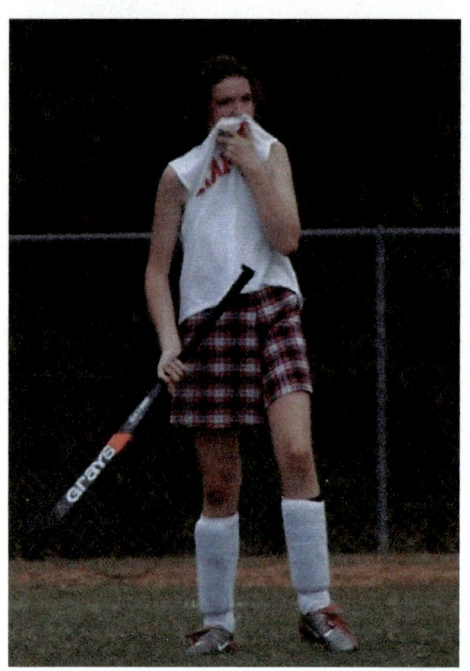

Meaghan during a field hockey game - 2005

Meaghan posing in the net for a school photo

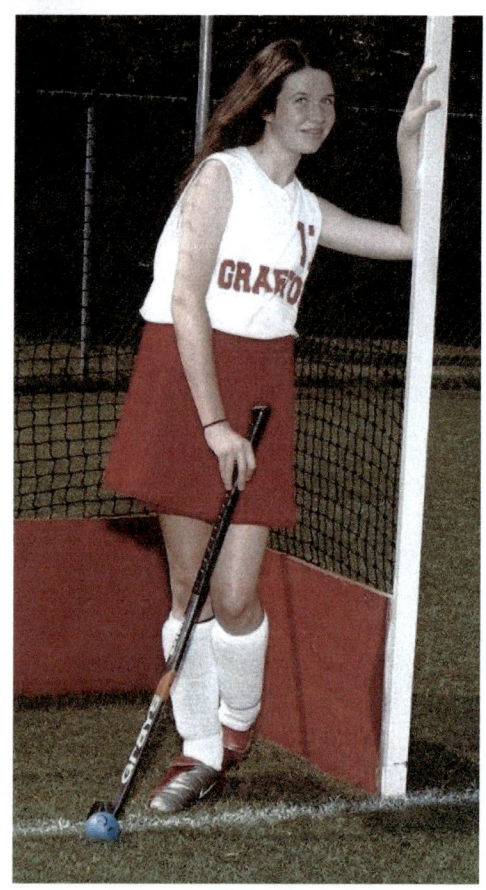

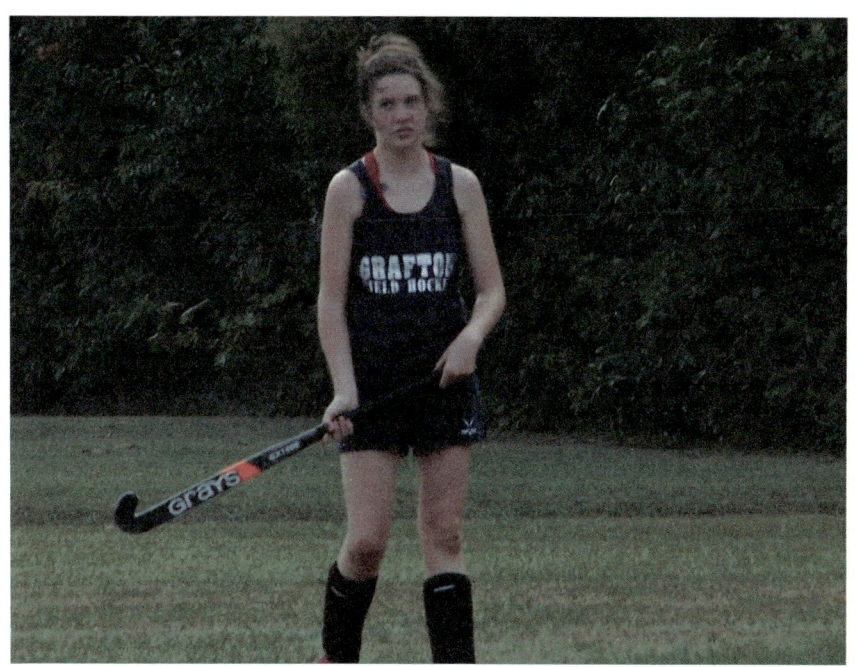

ABOVE: Meaghan - Summer of 2005

RIGHT: Fooling around on the sidelines

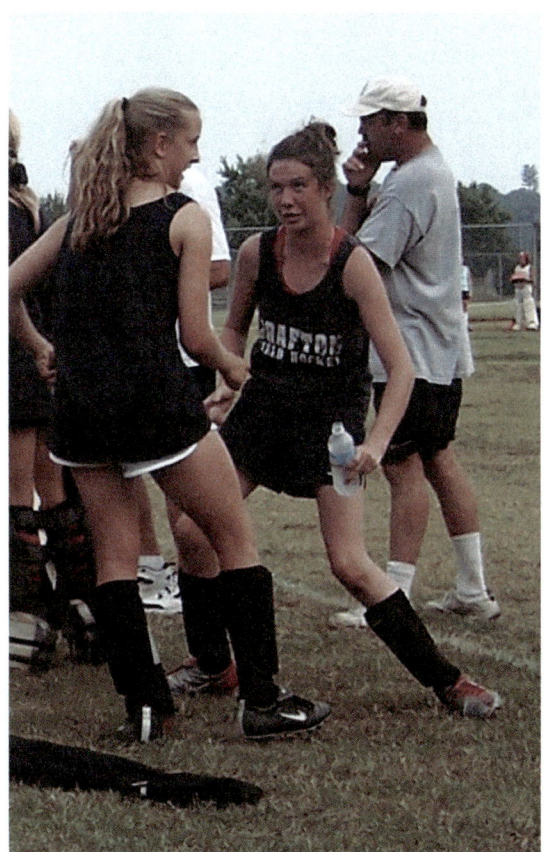

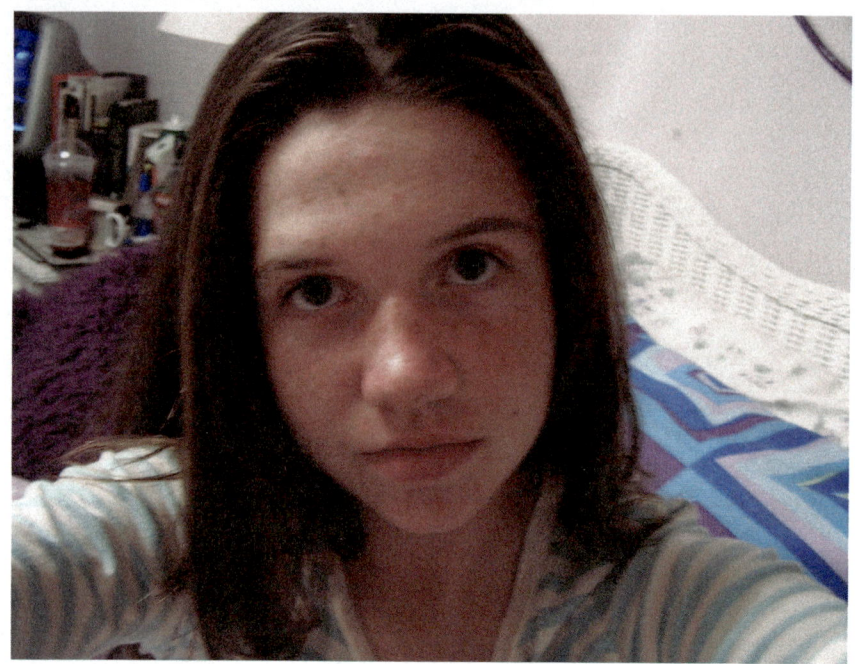

ABOVE: MySpace photo - 2004

BELOW: Gangsta MC Holla

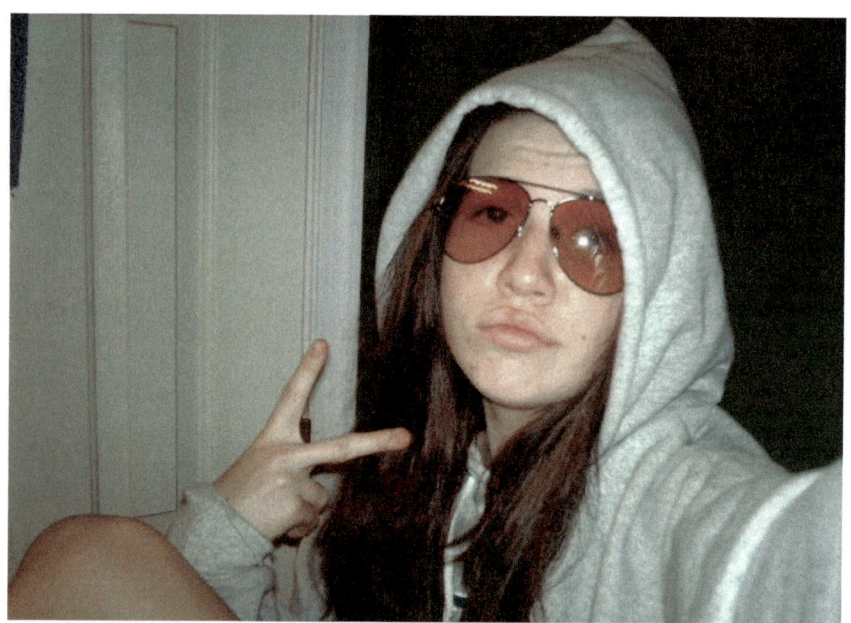

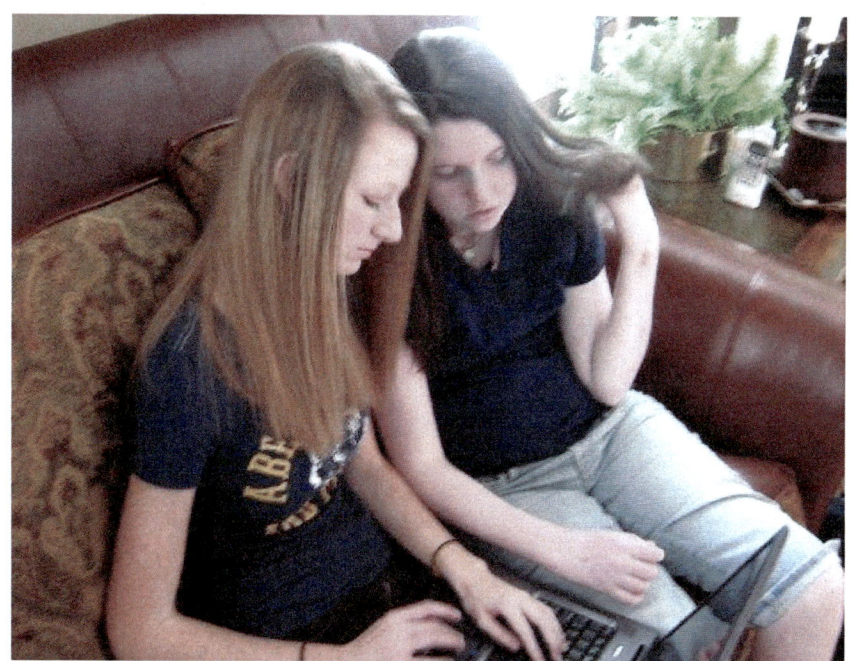

ABOVE: Meaghan and her best friend Katie work on projects for Students For a Cure on February 8, 2008. Meaghan would be admitted to CHKD later that day.

BELOW: Meaghan and her cousin Erin - February 2008

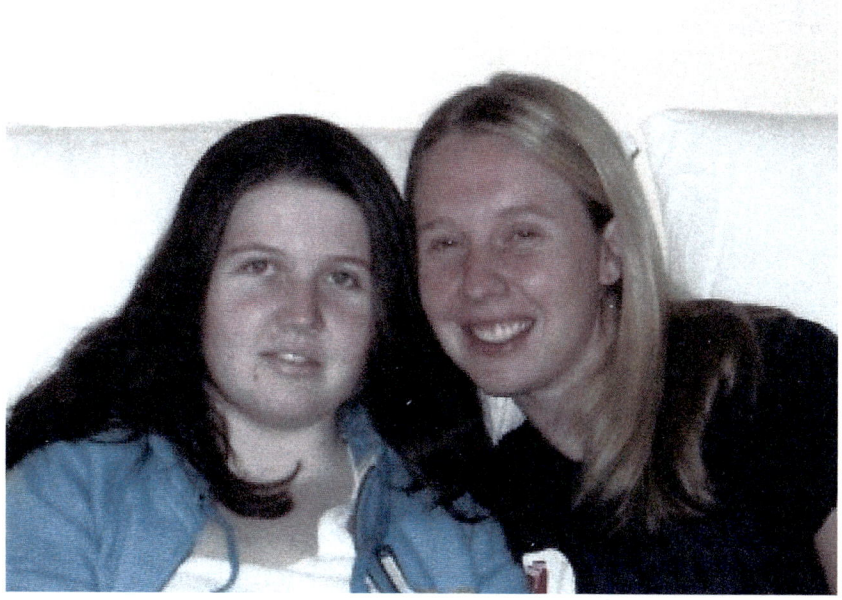

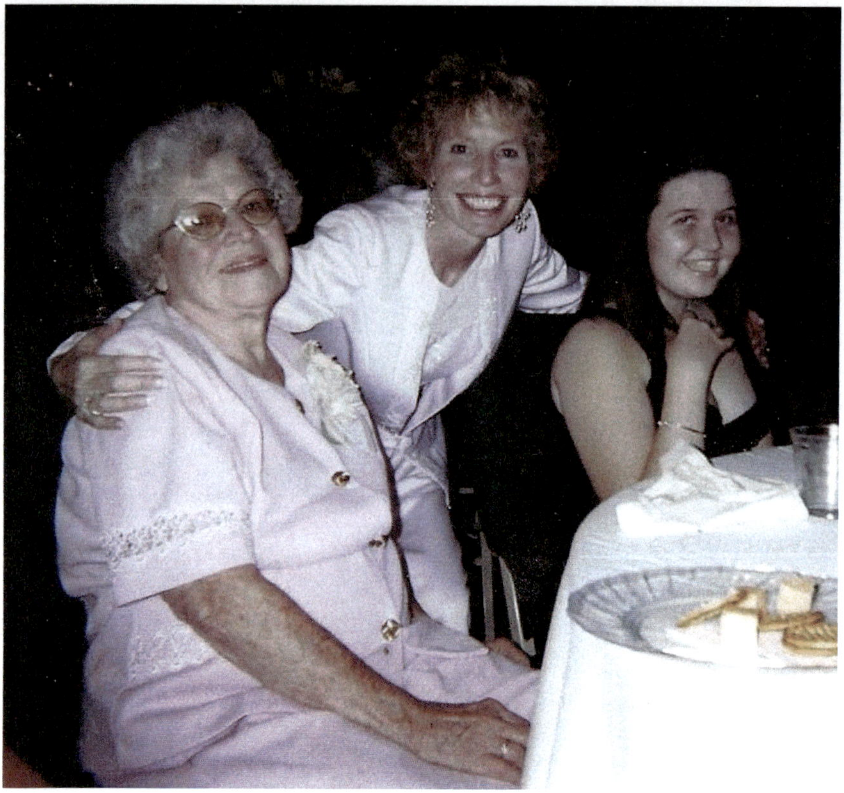

ABOVE: Meaghan, Karen, and Granda Burnham at Abbey's wedding in June of 2007

BELOW: Meaghan and Dad walk into her surprise 15th birthday party.

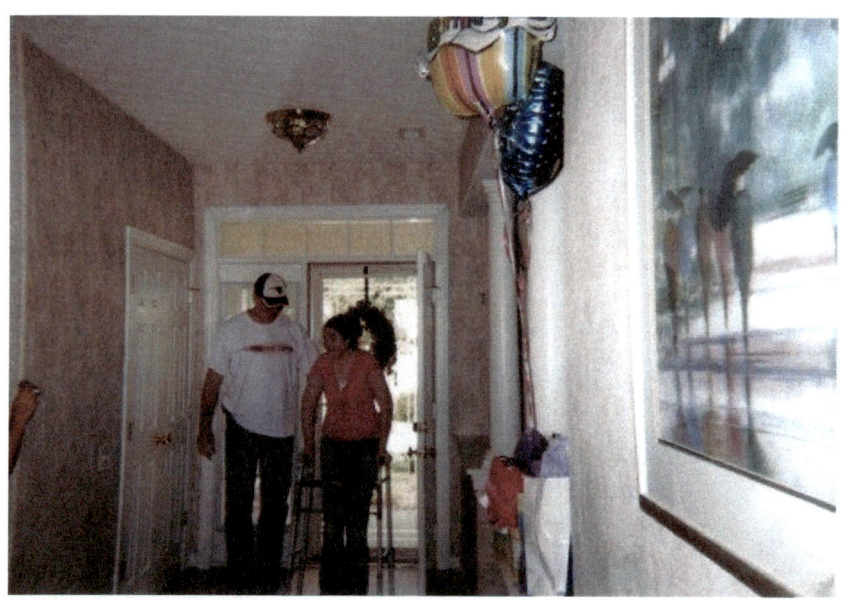

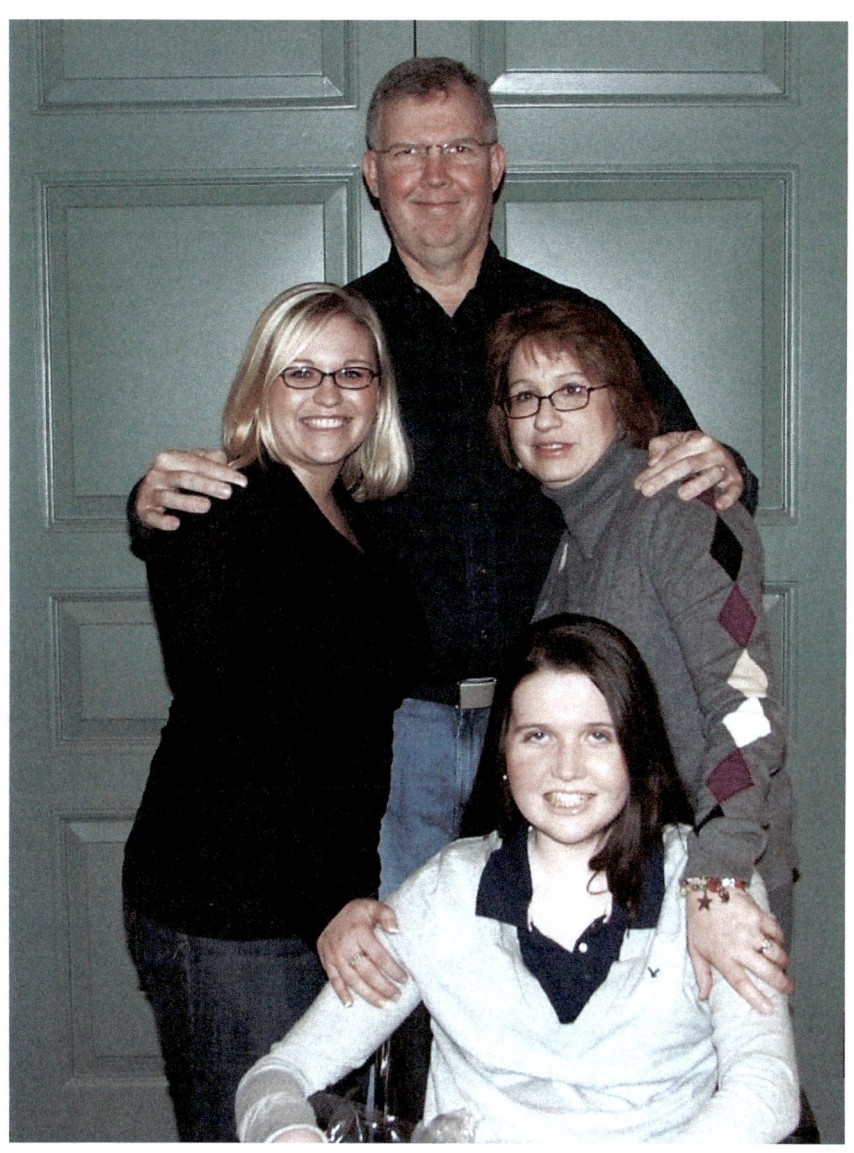

Meaghan with Mom, Dad, and cousin Jessica at the York County Courage Awards in February of 2008.

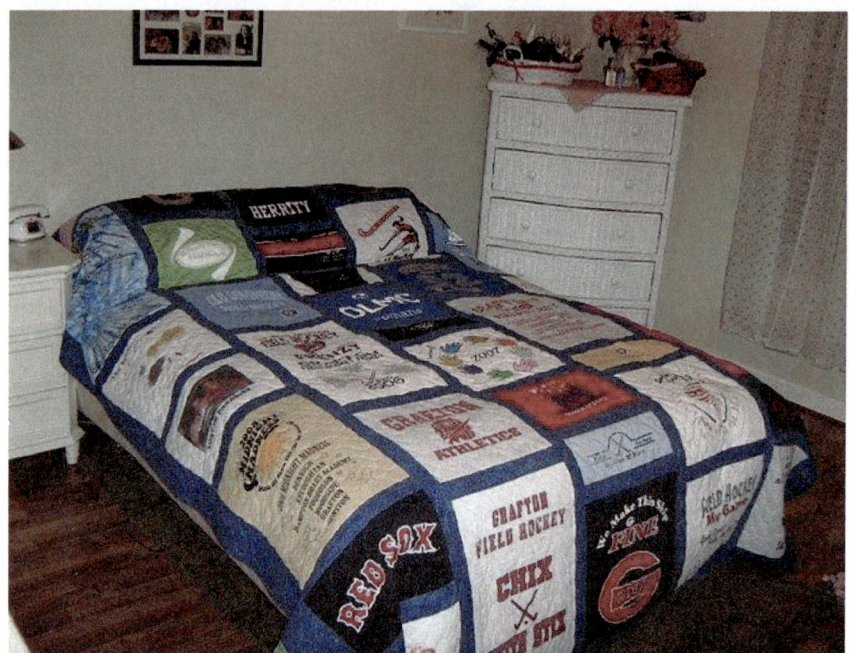

ABOVE: Quilt of Meaghan's life

BELOW: Homecoming 2007

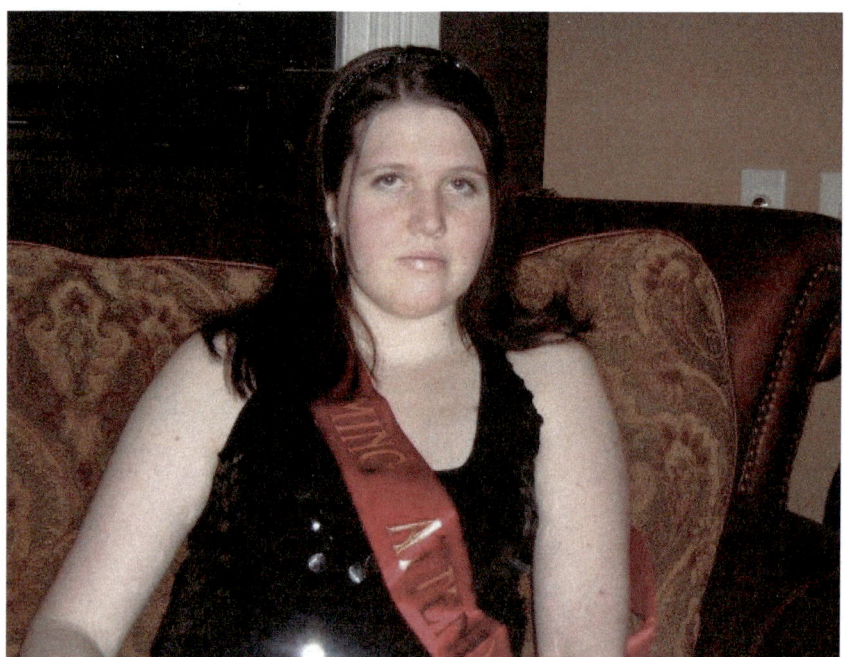

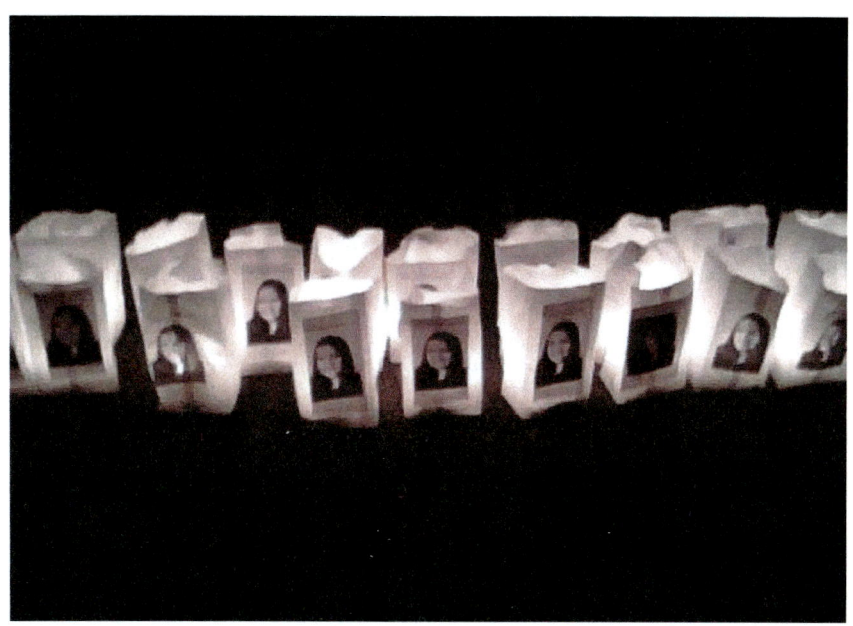

ABOVE: Relay for Life 2008

RIGHT: The Herrity family November 2007 - Meaghan, Janice, TJ, Jim, and Jimmy (photograph by Bill Manley of Flashes of Hope)

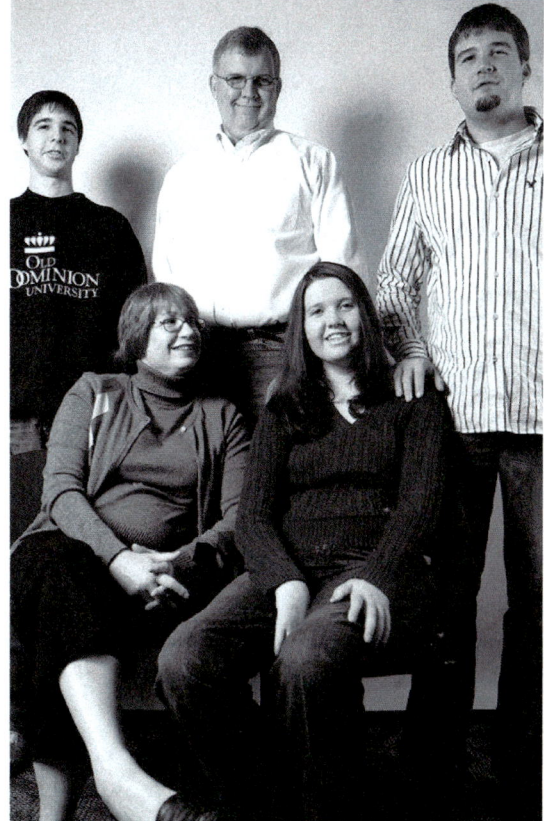

Chapter 10 – Losing Ground… But Not Hope

11,000 young people are diagnosed with cancer every year.

By the end of January, it was apparent that things were changing for the worse in Meaghan's body. At first the changes were subtle, but with each passing day it became more apparent that Meaghan was losing her battle with cancer. In addition to the headaches and blurred vision, Meaghan was having seizures several times a day. The lower half of her body clonused constantly, and repositioning her legs to distract the nerves no longer stopped the spasms. She also began to experience intense shooting pains throughout much of her body. She was often too physically weak to leave her bed.

Meaghan began to have difficulty swallowing and often choked on food, liquids, and medication, which I knew meant that the tumor had now reached areas that were once cancer free in the cervical area of her spine. To everyone's amazement, Meaghan rarely complained. She lived each day to its fullest with joy, purpose, contentment, and humor. I believe that Meaghan sensed that her time on this earth was coming to an end and wanted to make a difference in the lives of other children suffering from cancer before she died.

She formed a club at her high school and named it "Students For A Cure." Its mission was to raise both money and awareness for pediatric cancer patients and research. Meaghan hoped that through the efforts of the club, she and other students could help other children suffering from this awful disease. Although it was never her intention, through her selfless actions, she taught her peers to think of others before themselves.

On February eighth, a Saturday, Meaghan arranged a meeting with her friends at our home to begin plans for a fundraiser for St. Baldrick's. (St. Baldrick's is a national organization that raises both awareness and money for pediatric cancer research.) Meaghan was unusually weak that morning, and we tried to persuade her to postpone her meeting until the following day, but she was determined to have her meeting and directed Jim and me to get supplies and food. I helped Meaghan get ready and told her that her skin color was the best I had seen in weeks and that she looked absolutely radiant.

Janice Herrity

My happiness turned out to be short lived when Meaghan asked for an extra dose of morphine soon after taking the first. I knew at that moment that something was terribly wrong. Before I could get a chance to discuss the reason that she wanted additional morphine, her friends arrived and I dropped the subject. I watched Meaghan closely throughout the meeting. She was fully animated and engaged. There was no outward indication that she was in terrible pain. The group finalized plans for the St. Baldrick's fundraiser and then organized a book and video drive for both Edmarc and the oncology floor at CHKD. The meeting lasted a few hours and once the last girl left, Meaghan asked both Jim and me to assist her to her room and then told me that her pain was unbearable and that she needed another dose of morphine. I called Edmarc and was instructed to give Meaghan a third dose of morphine and to call back in two hours and report if the additional dose lessened her pain. Meaghan told us that the extra morphine did not ease her pain and that the pain was constant and excruciating. I was instructed to give her another dose, the fourth in an eight-hour period. It didn't help either, so we were told to take her to the ER. The Edmarc nurse would notify the oncologist on duty that Meaghan would be coming in.

Meaghan was so weak that she could not sit in her wheelchair, so Jim carried her to the van. I sat next to her in the car, and I could hear her whimpering in pain. My heart was ripped out by the sound; I was helpless to fix what was broken inside my little girl. On the way to the hospital, we all made polite conversation, avoiding the scenario that we each knew was about to unfold.

Once we arrived at CHKD, the ER personnel accessed Meaghan's port, drew blood, gave her additional pain meds, and then ordered an MRI. Once Meaghan was inside the MRI room, Jim and I talked for the first time since she had asked for additional morphine hours earlier. I told him that I knew that the scans were going to show disease progression. I also told him that that was the reason I had declined the MRI two weeks earlier. I was hoping to get another dose of chemotherapy and buy her time to restart the Avastin. Jim asked me why I didn't tell him this sooner, and I replied that I was simply hoping to be wrong and didn't want to share my fears.

Since Meaghan was out of sight, I began to cry. She hated seeing us cry, so we tried to never shed tears in front of her. I still can remember falling to the floor sobbing and then of course I began to vomit. It was 5:00am, and everything in the hospital, including the bathrooms, was locked, so I was throwing up in trash bins in the hallway. (I still wondered why security didn't escort me out. I guess the paper visitor badge had more influence than I ever imagined, or the security guards were all asleep on the job.)

Meaghan's Story

When I returned to the MRI waiting room, the technicians were just finishing up and taking the scans over to Norfolk General for analysis, which is never a good sign, especially on a Sunday morning. Since we expected that it would be a few hours before we got the results of the MRI, Meaghan and Jim insisted that I go out to the van and get some sleep and try to get the vomiting under control.

Within minutes, Jim was pounding on the van door frantically. The results of the MRI were back, and the surgeon who had initially operated on Meaghan had been called in to look at the scans to see if there was a possible surgical option. He told both Jim and Meaghan that there was nothing more that he could do.

I sat there stunned as Jim told me that the tumor that had shrunk two months earlier was now the entire length of both the cervical and thoracic sections of Meaghan's spine and that there were over twenty satellite tumors in the lumbar region. I immediately threw up and asked if Meaghan knew the results. Jim said, "Yes. She is completely calm, but she wants you." Once in the ER, I saw Meaghan and the first thing that she said was, "Mom are you feeling any better?" Unbelievably, she was worried about me! Meaghan was as Jim reported, completely composed and unruffled by the information. I then went to find the surgeon and see the scans myself. I took one look at the scans and turned around and returned to Meaghan. There was nothing to discuss. I had seen enough MRI scans over the past two years that I didn't need an explanation.

On the way back to Meaghan's room, I saw the oncology social worker. She had been called in to help us understand Meaghan's medical situation. She explained that the plan was to have Meaghan admitted to the oncology floor for a few days until we sorted through the information and could discuss the MRI results with her oncologist. She asked how Meaghan was handling the news, and I replied that she was completely composed and eerily peaceful. We told Meaghan at the beginning of this nightmare that we would always be honest with her and never withhold information to protect her, and I think that treating her as an adult and allowing her to have a voice in her medical treatment helped her to prepare both mentally and emotionally for this moment. Meaghan had always been aware that although she had beaten the initial odds, GBM's are very hard to kill and that if Ironitecan could not contain the tumor alone, the outcome would likely not be good.

Jim was with the oncologist on duty. They were on the phone with the oncologist at Duke looking for treatment options, and Jim was beginning to send out informative emails to hospitals all over the country to see if they had a new drug or a study that might help Meaghan. I asked Meaghan if she wanted to talk privately with the social worker about her scans. She replied, "No. I'm okay... but I feel like I've fallen into the deep end of a gigantic pool, and I'll have to swim with all my might to the shallow end to beat this." I looked at her and said, "That's a great metaphor, but you're not that great of a swimmer." Meaghan looked at me and said, "Duh, that's my point – it's the fight of my life."

Meaghan was adamant that she get some decent clothing for her hospital stay. She insisted that I return to Yorktown to get her clothes because Jim is somewhat "fashion impaired." Since I was in no condition to drive, Jim called Jimmy to drive me. When Jimmy arrived, he was completely frenzied and immediately went to see Meaghan. Within minutes of his arrival, Meaghan began insulting him because he was hung over, reeked of stale beer, had not showered, and smelled like an ashtray. They began to fight as if nothing was wrong. Jim and I didn't try to stop them because fighting with each other was normal and seemed to relieve the tension in the room.

Jimmy and I left a few minutes later. Our first stop was to find TJ and take him to the hospital so he could keep Meaghan company while Jim tried to reach anyone in the brain tumor community for advice and assistance. It was around 7:30 when we reached TJ's dorm, and the main door was locked. Jimmy's student ID did not allow him access to the dorm. When we buzzed to get in, no one answered. We waited outside until a student exited the building and grabbed the door and went in.

Once inside, we realized that we didn't know what TJ's room number was. We found the RA on duty, explained the situation, and had her open his door. I shook TJ awake and his first words were, "Oh my God, is Meaghan dead?" I said, "No" and then gave him the shortened version of what was happening and asked his roommate to take TJ to the hospital to save us a trip. TJ quickly dressed and grabbed his book bag and computer. He had a paper due the next day and said that he needed to finish it.

Jimmy then informed me that he also had a paper due the following day, so he would stay home, commute to school, and take care of the dogs. I still remember yelling at both of them about always waiting to the last minute to write their papers. I also yelled about other random things that irritated me about the two of them and about men in general. They both just stared at me and asked in unison if I needed professional help, or at least medication, because I was acting insane. I am still not sure if that was out of concern or an indiscriminate shot, because I was too weak to retaliate.

On the drive home, my cell phone started ringing. I was getting calls asking about Meaghan's condition. I was confused about how anyone knew that Meaghan was back in the hospital, but I quickly learned that Meaghan had posted on Facebook and Caringbridge that she was once

Meaghan's Story

again admitted to CHKD (she had omitted the details). Her friends had asked their parents to call me for information because many had seen her the day before and she had looked great. Out of respect for Meaghan's privacy I also omitted the details but told them that Meaghan's situation was "not good."

I asked a friend if she would call the high school Monday morning to see if we could get Meghan's class ring early because I was afraid that Meaghan might not be around for the ceremony later that month. My friend was stunned to hear me say those words because that was a place I did not go; I was always very optimistic to the outside world about Meaghan's condition and rarely shared my thoughts with anyone. My friend called the varsity field hockey coach and asked him to speak to the school principal and have her contact the ring company the following day. The coach did not want to wait until Monday to honor my request, so he called the junior class advisor to see if she could assist in getting Meaghan's ring early. The junior class advisor decided that she did not want to wait until Monday either, so she went to the high school to get the company's phone number, called the company representative, explained Meaghan's situation, and the company representative agreed to meet her at his office in Richmond.

The junior class advisor drove to Richmond, and the company representative found Meaghan's ring and gave it to her. She offered to pay the balance due on the ring, but the representative would not accept payment and told her that it was a gift from the ring company. She then drove back to Yorktown and met the coach at the high school. He then drove to the hospital to present Meaghan with her class ring that very evening! It was a complete surprise. Meaghan was so delighted that she showed the ring to every nurse and doctor that came into her room.

By evening, a steady stream of visitors had come to the hospital. Meaghan had a great visit with her friends. Laughter and silliness filled her room. She did not reveal the extent of her disease or the probable outcome. Nevertheless, her friends knew that the situation was serious and each one left her room with solemn expressions on their faces. While Meaghan's friends went to visit her, their parents stayed to comfort Jim and me. Our demeanor confirmed their fears – We were barely functioning. I was still vomiting, and he and TJ, for lack of a better word, were silent and shell shocked. The situation was incomprehensible. It was every parent's worst nightmare.

The next day we met with the oncologist. Jim and I (now the experts on this disease) had a list of clinical trials that might work, and we informed the doctor that we intended to pursue any and every practical solution. He told us he had "feelers" out to many institutions in the country and had spoken with the oncologists at both Dana-Farber and

Duke. Regrettably, he did not have any encouraging news to share. He said that they would continue to look into treatment options but that nothing looked promising.

He then spoke with us about "time and the quality of life" versus experimental treatments that would make Meaghan even sicker and may not even work. He also told us that we needed to consider signing a Do Not Resuscitate (DNR) order. He said that we did not have to make any decisions that day, but we needed to consider his advice and recommendations. We thanked him for his honesty. Meaghan loved him and we certainly trusted him, but this was our child, and we weren't ready to stop looking for a new treatment. Meaghan was adamant that she see her MRI scans, and her oncologist agreed.

He had her come downstairs to the clinic to view them and said he wanted to talk to her alone to answer any questions she might have. From where we were standing, we could see Meaghan pointing to the large areas of white on the scan. She asked the doctor if he had a chemotherapy that would work for her, and he said that he hadn't found anything yet. She also asked him if she was going to die, and he said, "Yes." Her reply was, "Okay."

She then asked that Jim and I come to join them. We had nothing left to discuss, so we stood near Meaghan in silence. She was completely composed and stoic; there was not a tear, no anger, and no fear. Meaghan then asked us to take her back upstairs because her oncologist had other kids that needed him. She reminded him to continue to look for a new chemotherapy and said that she didn't even care if she lost her hair this time.

Upstairs, Meaghan remained peaceful. She talked on the phone, did some homework, chatted on the computer, ate dinner, showered, and encouraged Jim to go home to sleep for the night. Jim had been in the same clothes since Saturday night and had been taking catnaps in the van in the CHKD parking lot, so he reluctantly agreed. He left around eleven and told me to call him if anything changed. He said that he would be back immediately.

Meaghan fell asleep soon afterward. I was unable to sleep, so I sat next to her and held her hand. Around two in the morning, the nurse came to give Meaghan her medication. This was not unusual, but that night was different. Meaghan began to choke on the medication and had a seizure. The nurse called for help and within seconds, several oncology nurses came to assist. She also paged the doctor on call to come to Meaghan's room immediately. Meaghan was having difficulty breathing. Machines were beeping, the nurses were suctioning her throat, and nothing they were doing was helping her catch her breath. The

Meaghan's Story

nurses must have called some sort of code, because interns arrived just to observe. I had spent enough time in a hospital to know that that was not a good thing. This situation had a lot in common with the day that the boy died in the clinic.

I was asked to step away from Meaghan so the nurses could get the situation under control. I called Jim, and once he heard the chaos in the background, he knew that the situation was unusual and said that he would be there shortly. The episode, whatever it was, lasted for about twenty minutes. Eventually Meaghan stopped choking and began to breathe normally, and the color returned to her face. The medical explanation was that the tumor was pressing on a nerve or muscle or something - no one knew what the exact cause was. The "episode" was a new development in an ever-changing situation. Once order was restored and Meaghan and I were alone, she looked at me and said, "I refused to die before Dad's birthday (February twenty-first), and I wasn't going tonight." Jim showed up a few minutes later, and she told him the same thing. We sat there stunned and held her hand as she fell back to sleep.

The next day we signed the DNR with tears rolling down our faces. Seeing Meaghan fight to breathe was more than I could endure. Jim and I knew that it was necessary. The oncologist placed the form in with Meaghan's orders and told us that if another episode occurred, the hospital personnel would not attempt heroic matters to save her life. We then learned that we would need to have a second DNR for home as well. Lesson XXI: it is Virginia law that if anyone passes away at home without a DNR, your home becomes a crime scene. Family members are separated and interviewed until emergency personnel reach a conclusion. We were informed that even though we had a DNR, we could still call 911 to revive Meaghan as it was our always our decision, but the DNR would eliminate police, fire, and ambulance on the street and would ultimately protect us.

When I pressed the nurse about what we needed protection from, we were told that parents have been known to kill their terminally ill children (this information absolutely stunned us both). The nurse then explained that with a DNR at home, all we would need to do when Meaghan passed away was to call Edmarc. The Edmarc nurse would then come to our home and "pronounce," therefore eliminating the bedlam and chaos. We never discussed the DNR order with Meaghan or the boys. The choice we made was made out of love and respect for our daughter, and it was the hardest decision of our lives.

The next day Meaghan was discharged from CHKD. Before she could leave, she needed to get a morphine pump that would be attached to her at all times for pain management. Jim and an aide took Meaghan to the van, and I went to sign the discharge orders. The nurse gave me prescriptions to fill for breakthrough pain, seizures, and just about any other medical crisis that might occur. As her primary caregiver, I was given instructions on what to do and whom to call for each scenario.

As I was going through each scenario with the nurse, tears flowed, and my heart ached. I was terrified that I would fail in my care for Meaghan and ultimately cause her greater harm. Leaving the hospital that day was oddly reminiscent of bringing home a newborn. I was given instructions, phone numbers, and prescriptions, but I had no idea what to expect.

Jim and Meaghan were waiting for me in front of the hospital and could not imagine what was taking me so long. They assumed that I was chatting with the staff or that I was at the gift shop. Only when I got into the car and Jim saw the prescriptions and teaching material did he understand what took me so long. I told Jim that we needed to stop at the pharmacy on the way home and then dropped the matter. When the pharmacist saw my list of prescriptions, he just looked at me and said, "Oh, I'm sorry. We'll fill these at once."

A whole new world was unraveling - one that I wished did not exist. We were out of options, and CHKD had basically told us to go home and wait for Meaghan to die. Meaghan had been told a year earlier, after her first reoccurrence, that there was a real chance that she would not make it. But this time was different – every medical professional had come to the same conclusion. How our world had changed in just four short days...

Chapter 11 – Waiting for a Miracle

I left the pharmacy with seven new prescriptions, and before I could even read the directions, the home delivery pharmacy arrived with all of Meaghan's IV medications and supplies. I would have to learn to administer those as well. The situation was surreal; we were out of medical options, and now my job was essentially to manage Meaghan's pain, keep her comfortable, and wait either for a miracle or the end. Jim and I were literally frozen with fear, but we knew that inaction, doubt, and self-pity would not help Meaghan, so we chose to adjust – not accept – our new world.

Meaghan, on the other hand, was calm and looking forward to a group visit from her friends. That evening around thirty of her friends came over to welcome her home. Meaghan sat in the living room and other than the tubing that attached to the morphine pump, there was no outward sign of the seriousness of her medical condition. She did not discuss her illness, and neither did her friends. The conversation was that of typical teen talk – school, SAT's, car accidents, clothing, and *Grey's Anatomy*.

I still remember watching her – animated and laughing, completely composed, and smiling from ear to ear in spite of the news that she had been given less than twenty-four hours earlier. I sat in another room making polite conversation with her friend's parents. Jim went into the office, frantically searching for a new therapy to beat the cancer. We knew that there was nothing available in the United States, so he was sending emails to hospitals and research institutes all over the world. We were keenly aware that our insurance wouldn't pay for treatment outside the US; nevertheless we both were prepared to sell everything we owned, mortgage our future, and take Meaghan to Timbuktu if she had a chance of beating the cancer.

I never felt as frightened as I did that first night. I knew that Meaghan's condition was grave, and as her main caregiver I was her first line of defense in the event of a medical emergency. I was absolutely terrified that I would not be able to remember the nurse's instructions.

Meaghan and I talked that night about the very real possibility that she might die within the next few weeks. She told me that she completely understood her situation and that she was okay with any outcome. She paraphrased Karen's sentiments and said, "If a miracle comes, I'll be healed; if not, I'll go to Heaven – it's a win-win situation." Then in a matter of fact tone she asked to turn on Law & Order – SVU and said, "I sleep like a baby after watching a good rape" and burst into laughter.

Janice Herrity

As bleak as the situation was, we were not without hope that a miracle was on its way. That gave us the strength to get through that night and the following months. I suppose it is the human spirit that sustains us during the most desperate of situations and gives us the courage and strength to face tomorrow. As I mentioned before, we were straddling two worlds – the world of hope and the world of stark reality. We chose the world of hope, and that choice would sustain us until the very end.

The next few days we continued life as we had come to know it. Meaghan continued with her routine of school and therapy, never wavering. The boys stayed at school because we felt that they needed to remain as normal as possible in this situation. We had learned that panic and fear were counterproductive, and Meaghan didn't want them to stop their lives for her. Jim chose not to return to DC to work but chose to telecommute from the house. I was amazed that he could focus, but he did.

We could no longer sugarcoat Meaghan's illness to our families. We told them that Meaghan was most likely going to die within the next few weeks, so if they wanted to visit her, they should come soon. My family chose not to come, and I was thankful. I did not think that my eighty-two year old parents could handle seeing their youngest grandchild in such a debilitated condition.

Jim's sister and her family, including Erin, decided that they wanted to see Meaghan and flew in for a weekend visit. I felt comfortable knowing that Meaghan was in Erin's capable hands and I napped for the first time in days. Meaghan loved seeing them and had a wonderful time visiting. Around seven that evening, Meaghan showed signs of exhaustion, so they returned to their hotel.

That evening when I gave Meaghan her nine o'clock medications, She began to have some difficulty breathing and started to drift in and out of consciousness. I immediately called Edmarc, and the nurse on duty came at once. Meaghan was only taking five breathes per minute, and she kept telling us that there was a man standing at the edge of her bed watching her - this is not unusual when the end is near, according to hospice personnel. Jim called the boys and asked them to come home and then called Erin and asked that she come back to assist the Edmarc nurse. Meaghan's breathing was becoming increasing shallow, and she became less coherent with each passing hour. Both nurses were sure that Meaghan would not make it through the night and suggested that we say our goodbyes. Jim then called his sister and asked her to return to the house, and he phoned our parish priest.

The Edmarc nurse told us that children hang on to protect their parents and suggested that we have a heart to heart talk with

Meaghan's Story

Meaghan and give her permission to die. It was the hardest thing we have ever had to do – an experience that I would not wish upon my worst enemy. There are no words to describe the anguish and heartache that we felt as we told our precious daughter that it was okay to die and held her as she fought to breathe. Jim and I told Meaghan how proud we were of her and that we loved her with all our hearts. We told Meaghan that she had enriched our lives and that she would always be in our thoughts and hearts. We told her that we admired her strength, her courage, and her tenacity. We told her that she need not stay in this world for us and that in time we would be okay. We gave Meaghan permission to die.

We both knew that we would never be whole again, but Meaghan needed to hear us say that we would move forward with life and not be bitter. But truthfully, how can a parent ever completely recover from outliving their child?

Around three in the morning, our parish priest arrived and immediately went to Meaghan's room. We all prayed, and the priest made the sign of the cross on Meaghan's forehead and began the Sacrament of Healing. Meaghan promptly opened her eyes and said, "That better not be Last Rites because I'm not going anywhere before February twenty-second!" He looked at her and said, "I know - you tell me that every time I visit you," and she began to laugh hysterically.

Over the next few hours Meaghan's breathing returned to normal, and she fell asleep. When she awoke the next morning her first words were "Good Morning America… I'm still here!" She then requested her computer because she needed to see if American Eagle had any new clothes on their website. She asked me to order a dress from the website for her to be buried in. I asked her why she wanted that dress, as it wasn't particularly special - just a simple sundress. Meaghan then remarked that she wanted to choose the dress she was to be buried in "because she was afraid that I might dress her like a slut!"

I looked at her and said, "I didn't realize that was a problem." I added that if she didn't behave, I would throw out all her old clothes, because they were obviously too slutty, and replace them with a new wardrobe made entirely of gingham and ruffles! She mumbled her response, "Well played, mother … checkmate."

She then showed me a poem that she had written and dedicated to my sister Karen. Although she said that the poem was about Karen, it was apparent that it was semi-autobiographical. As I read her poem, Meaghan's words touched my heart and gave me a sense of peace. She had been ill for almost two years and had grown from a scared teenager into a beautiful self-assured young woman. She never wavered in her faith and showed no sign of fear of the journey ahead of her.

Janice Herrity

The Sunrise from the Window

Meaghan Herrity

Dedicated to: Karen B. Aldrich

The sun is sinking into the horizon
Soon it will be dark and the night air will come
It will be too chilly for her to be outside
Sitting, bundled beneath blankets, in an old wooden deck chair
Watching the waves crash against the jetties
And smiling to herself as children laugh and play in the distance.

This is her routine, when she wakes
She musters what little strength she has left
Dresses herself, refusing help from anyone
Pours a cup of coffee, and limps out to the deck
Finds her favorite chair and sips her coffee
Watching and waiting for the world to awake.

From the deck she can see everything and everyone
When neighbor's pass by her, she always waves, musters a 1000-watt smile
Occasionally she'll engage in a conversation, if she has the strength
If not, her eyes drop apologetically as she fades to sleep mid-sentence
When she wakes, she'll ask for water and her dog-eared, tattered Bible
I just can't comprehend the affliction placed upon our family.

Never once did she complain, and rarely shed a tear
Even when the incomprehensible news was told, that awoke us from our nightmare
And made us feel like small children awaking in the night
Searching for someone to hold and comfort them

Meaghan's Story

Chase the demons away, and make it alright

Yet as hard as we tried, we couldn't chase the demons away, we had no way to make it alright.

The doctors said that she was beyond repair, there was nothing left they could do

The cancer had spread, and they had no solution but for her to make herself comfortable

And wait for the inevitable end,

As if she was a broken toy that couldn't be fixed, tossed aside and forgotten

Every day, as long as the weather permits, she sits on the deck and waits for the end

No sign of fear is shown on her face as she watches the waves roll in.

And laughs as children run along the beach and build castles in the sand

She's become pale, thin, and too weak for much activity

Her face is pale, all of her hair has fallen out so she wears a knit cap to keep warm

Tubes are attached to every part of her body

To feed her, fill her lungs with pure oxygen and try to keep her alive

Just for another day, just for another day.

From where I stand in the kitchen, I can see her positioned in her rickety old chair

With her Bible placed in her lap, I watch as her lips move as she silently re-reads the passages

Words she's read countless times, words she still believes, for reasons I'll never know

I sit awake at night and wonder how this could have happened

To a woman who did all she could to try and make other's lives a bit easier

And welcomed others with open arms without judgment.

At night I sit in my room and sob silently, trying to comprehend why

Janice Herrity

My thoughts and tears keep me awake as I try to find a way to help

But, there is never a solution

It's bright outside and the temperature is warm with a slight breeze

Ideal weather, the sun is at a perfect angle in the sky which makes my surroundings feel brighter

Almost safer, as the trees sway in the wind and the ocean sparkles.

My mother notices me watching from the window and waves to me

I take this as a signal to join her and walk onto the deck and breathe in the sea air

Air that brings back memories of happier times long ago

When my mother and I frolicked in the surf and built castles in the sand

She sits in her chair and smiles as I pull up one of the plush, padded deck chairs we beg her to use

But she has a routine that does not include comfortable deck chairs.

Her cup of coffee is still full, it's been month's since she could drink it

Always though, she'll pour a cup, refusing to break her routine because of one little setback

Her pale frail hand squeezes my hand gently, and stares into my eyes for what seems like an eternity

When she lets go, she stares out at the ocean and sighs

Silently she picks up her Bible and begins to read.

I went to the kitchen in the morning

What I saw made time stand still, an empty whitewashed, rickety old chair

Dropping the glass of juice I'd been drinking

I listened to it shatter and stared at the shards of glass on the floor, frozen where I stood.

After seconds, minutes, maybe hours, I'll never be sure, I ran to her bedroom

She was there in her bed, eyes closed, a serene look on her face

Meaghan's Story

Her Bible was beside her, blankets were piled upon her pale, small frame
I noticed the sun rising as I glanced out the window, and realize she's gone
Rising up like the sun to a better place, ready to begin a new routine.

The days and weeks ahead would be filled with bittersweet moments. Meaghan was honored to be chosen the 2008 York County Outstanding Youth for Courage. The ceremony to honor exceptional high school students is held yearly in May, but because of Meaghan's declining health she was recognized alone at a Board of Supervisors meeting in February. We received a call from a county official congratulating Meaghan on her selection. Her name and story were submitted by the varsity field hockey coach at Grafton. He had several essays written by her friends detailing Meaghan's journey and how she had inspired them.

When we arrived for the ceremony, we were completely taken aback by the number of friends and teachers who came to witness Meaghan receive her award. She was humbled by their support. Meaghan looked absolutely radiant that evening, and other than her wheelchair and morphine pump hidden in a purse, she gave no indication to the outside world of how very ill she was.

The following day, Meaghan was confirmed in the Catholic Church. Because she was so ill, our parish priest and her youth minister came to the house to perform the sacrament. Meaghan chose the name Brigid, as her Confirmation name (St. Brigid is one of the patron saints of Ireland) to acknowledge her Irish ancestry, which was very important to her. Meaghan's English teacher was her sponsor, and several family friends also gathered to watch her officially join the Church. The Sacrament of Confirmation was extremely important to Meaghan, and she told me that it was something that she always wanted to do. She was delighted that she was able to complete that important step in her faith and insisted on a new outfit and a party afterwards to celebrate.

Meaghan's poem was featured in an upcoming Edmarc newsletter along with her York County Courage award and a few photos. Edmarc asked her to share her journey and thoughts. Here are her words:

> *When I awoke April 14, 2006 unable to walk, the last thing that I ever imagined was that I would be diagnosed with spinal cancer. I had just run four miles earlier that week with ease, even now, two years later, it is still inconceivable to me that both events could occur within days of one another. Once I learned I had cancer I knew I had two choices, I could either be a victim, bitter and angry, or I could fight and embrace the disease and life*

itself. I chose to fight; and have discovered that each day brings with it new challenges, but it also brings hope.

When I was first told I had cancer the advice I was given was, "To take it one day at a time." I can still remember rolling my eyes and thinking, "What do you know, you don't know me, and you don't have cancer." However, it has turned out to be the best advice I ever have gotten, and I have applied it to all aspects of my life. Having cancer is a scary experience. I know I could die, but I still have hope for a cure. I believe in miracles and see no reason why a miracle cannot happen for me, or for any other child. That is what I hold on to, that is what gets me through the tough days.

On my journey I realized that cancer can happen to anyone. I have seen children of all ages, races and ethnic backgrounds with this disease. Cancer is indiscriminate and it strikes without mercy or warning. Lives are turned upside down with the diagnosis, and often left in disrepair. I have seen children in hospitals without their parents because they had siblings to care for, or they needed to work to pay for health insurance, or pay the bills. I always considered myself lucky because my mother was able to be with me and I did not have to face the disease and treatment alone.

My new life as a teenager with cancer involved never ending doctor visits, chemotherapy, drug cocktails, radiation, pain management, occupational, and physical therapy, as well as keeping up with my studies to graduate on time with my class. I left my "typical teenage" life behind and focused all my energy on walking again and beating cancer. I thought I had beaten it, but in February 2007, my bimonthly MRI showed a spot had reoccurred. By the time a new treatment came, the spot was six centimeters. The new treatment stopped the growth and the tumor even shrank, until February 2008 when it reoccurred a second time.

Presently, there is not a chemotherapy that will work for me, but my parents continue to look daily for studies and talk with other brain tumor patients and parents online to exchange ideas. I have begun acupuncture along with Chinese herbal medicines to see if that helps, and I do feel better and look forward to the treatments. I am on numerous prayer lists throughout the United States, and I am not giving up hope for a miracle.

I am sixteen years old and I do not believe it is my time to go, so I will continue to fight, until I decide it is time to stop. I have *chosen to fight with actions and began to organize with my friends fundraisers for St. Baldrick's, Relay for Life, and CHKD. We sold chocolates at my high school to raise money for St. Baldrick's, and had a new and gently used book and video drive for 8B. The outpouring of support from family, friends, doctors, nurses, other patients and their families, and my personal faith has given me the strength and courage to continue daily to fight this awful disease and to become cancer free. My plan is to fulfill my goal of walking as a survivor at the 2009 Relay for Life in Yorktown, and to walk across the stage at my high school graduation, go to college, and help other children beat this disease.*

The following week was Jim's birthday, and we were all uncertain what would unfold once the day passed. Meaghan had told us numerous times that she wasn't going to die before February twenty-first and ruin his birthday for the rest of his life. Thankfully, the twenty-second came and went uneventfully. Over the next few weeks Meaghan finished her mandatory state testing, English term paper, and all school assignments and was inducted into the GHS National Honor Society. NHS inductions are usually held in May, but because of Meaghan's illness she was inducted early. We planned to go to the school for the ceremony, but Meaghan had a particularly bad day, so the induction ceremony was held in her room. She wore her pajamas.

Meaghan was once again honored and touched by the outpouring of love and support as her induction was witnessed by friends, peers, teachers and her principal. Meaghan joked that her attire may have been a first not only for the GHS chapter of the National Honor Society, but the entire NHS! She had us capture the moment with photos for posterity.

Each day, Meaghan began to encounter new health challenges. She was in continuous pain. Her eyesight and balance worsened, and she would seizure several times a day. She was unfazed by her ever-changing situation and simply went about the task of living, focusing on school and life as she had come to know it.

I'm a firm believer that the connections we make in this world are not by coincidence, but are part of the overall fabric of God's plan for us. This became increasingly evident when, by chance, our next-door neighbor's father, a renowned acupuncturist and Buddhist monk, visited to treat his son-in-law's knee problem. Our neighbor told her father about Meaghan, and he offered to come treat her as well. We were open to any treatment option and were thrilled by his generous offer.

The first night the doctor came to treat Meaghan, she was in tremendous pain. Her skin tone had a grayish tinge, and her breathing was a bit labored. The doctor quickly examined Meaghan, but before he began, he prayed and asked the spirits for guidance in placing the needles where they were most needed. He then proceeded to position the needles with great care. After all the needles were inserted, the doctor prayed once more and wrote words in Chinese which he taped above Meaghan's bed to "Bless her and ward off evil spirits." I joked that maybe we should have it made into wallpaper and put on every wall in the house. I guess my humor was lost in translation because when his daughter relayed my message, he just stared at me.

The doctor spoke very little English and used his daughter as a translator to communicate with Meaghan. She explained the procedure and asked Meaghan if she could feel it each time her father sited a needle. Unfortunately, Meaghan was unable to tell where the needles were being placed. Once again, she had lost feeling in many parts of her body. The next morning brought us hope that a miracle was indeed on its way when Meaghan awoke with the ability to wiggle her toes and lift both of her legs – things that she had not been able to do for weeks! Additionally, feeling had returned to numerous areas of Meaghan body, her skin was no longer gray, and she had an appetite for the first time in weeks – it was truly amazing. The doctor came over around eight that morning to check on Meaghan and was overjoyed to see her sitting up and eating. He then asked what her diet consisted of, and I replied that she was eating almost nothing. He was greatly concerned by her lack of appetite and instructed me to make Meaghan a combination of puréed rice, beef, and sesame seed oil. She was to eat the mixture at least twice a day. He said it would help with her digestion and would give Meaghan the nutrition her body was lacking. The concoction looked like mush, and smelled horrible, but Meaghan ate it and often asked for a second helping.

The doctor then physically examined Meaghan. When he saw her incision, he became very agitated. His daughter explained that he was upset because eastern medicine holds that cutting the body interferes with the flow of Chi. She explained that when people become stressed or ill, the body's Chi, or energy, becomes blocked. She went on to explain that acupuncture releases the bad energy so the good energy can flow naturally again. The doctor also suggested that we add Chinese herbs and medicine and stop all the western drugs that we were giving Meaghan. We told him that we respected his opinion but did not feel comfortable taking Meaghan off the drugs, especially the pain medication, but we did agree to add Chinese herbs and medication. The doctor needed to send to China to get the medicine. It cost twenty-five hundred dollars, but we had nothing to lose. It was a "Hail Mary." We were hoping and praying that the herbs were the miracle that we were looking for.

Meaghan's Story

The doctor came regularly for the next three weeks. After each acupuncture treatment, Meaghan's circulation, movement, and sensation to touch improved greatly.

The Month of March came and went, and our neighbor's father returned to Korea. Jim had to leave to begin a new contract in Miami. Meaghan looked fantastic and was beginning to lift her legs again with ease, and her pain once more began to subside. However, cancer is cruel and as quickly as Meaghan seemed to improve, her world took a turn for the worse. It became apparent that the tumor was not shrinking, and it began to effect parts of Meaghan's body that were previously unaffected. Meaghan awoke one morning unable to use her hands. She was not frantic but rather matter of fact about the whole situation. With an eerily calm demeanor she said, "I'm okay living my life in a wheelchair, but I've got to use my hands. Can you call Toni (Occupational Therapist) to see if she can come over today so I can begin working on getting the use of them back?"

Her words gave me the chills. I was very sure that, had this happened to me, I would not have her confidence or handle the situation with the same grace. Because the tumor affected the nerves that controlled Meaghan's fine and gross motor skills, she needed assistance dressing and feeding herself, and she began to use voice activated software for schoolwork. Although the tumor caused Meaghan to become a quadriplegic, she continued with occupational and physical therapy, never wavering from her goal of beating the disease.

The cancer was growing rapidly. Meaghan began to have tremendous difficulty swallowing, so I puréed all of her food. I also ground-up many of her pills and put the residue into a syringe with liquid and shot it down her throat to make sure that she got all of her medications.

For almost two years, I prayed each night that God would heal Meaghan. But after she became a quadriplegic, my prayers changed. I still continued to pray for a miracle, but I asked God to take Meaghan peacefully in her sleep if the miracle that we were so desperately seeking was not coming. Watching a loved one slowly deteriorate is absolutely unbearable, and as a mother, not being able to fix my daughter's situation was insufferable. But I never gave up hope that a miracle was coming, and neither did Meaghan.

Even through all the chaos, Meaghan continued to awaken each day with a smile on her face and with a determination to make each moment she had on this earth meaningful. Meaghan was not in denial about her disease, and we talked daily about her probable outcome. She gave me a to do list and asked me to write this book alone and let the world know that she was more than an entry in a medical journal that read, "Fourteen year-old female, spinal glioblastomia, died two years after initial diagnosis." Meaghan said she wanted the world to know who she was and how she lived. She wanted the world to know about her sense of purpose and her spirit, and that she was happy despite her illness.

She asked me to continue to raise money for the charities that had helped us during her illness, especially Edmarc, and to buy myself a Mercedes. I unenthusiastically agreed, knowing she was getting her last thoughts in order.

The vow that I had made to myself in ICU two years earlier (that Meaghan's dignity would never be compromised) was tested daily. She was so weak that it took three people to move her into her wheelchair, and bathing became a nightmare for both logistical and safety reasons. The logical solution would have been to give Meaghan a sponge bath in bed, but Meaghan and I chose the emotional response. Together we devised a plan that allowed her to have a bath and wash her hair each day. Our plan worked beautifully. Each day I would disconnect her from the morphine pump and give her an oral dose of morphine to manage her pain, dress her in a string bikini, and cover her port with saran wrap, gauze, and tape to keep it dry. I would then ask whoever was assisting (on weekdays the aides, and on weekends Jim and the boys) to help me get Meaghan into a sitting position and then transfer her to the wheelchair. The tumor had affected Meaghan's balance, so we would belt her in the wheelchair. We then maneuvered the wheelchair into the bathroom and two of us would lift her into the bath chair and belt her in. After ten minutes we would reverse the procedure, always mindful of the tumor, trying to avoid any additional pain.

As the following days unfolded, things began to get even worse. Meaghan woke up one morning unable to speak above a whisper. We hoped that it was her asthma kicking in due to the change of seasons, but this was not the case. She had developed both pneumonia and strep throat. The doctor ordered antibiotics but warned that her immune system was so weakened by the cancer that this time she may not recover. The hospice nurse suggested that I call Jim and the boys to come home because the situation was so grave. I then called the mother of one of Meaghan's best friends to inform her of Meaghan's condition.

She went to the high school to take her daughter out of school so she could see Meaghan one last time. Within a few hours, word had spread throughout the high school, and about forty of Meaghan's friends left school and gathered by Meaghan's side to say their goodbyes. By the time Jim and the boys returned home, Meaghan's voice had returned and her lungs were clear. The nurse was stunned because hours earlier Meaghan had pneumonia in both lungs, and her throat was covered in pustules. I cannot say if her "cure" was the result of the antibiotics, or a higher power who gave us some extra time, but it was nothing short of miraculous.

As I mentioned numerous times before, cancer is both unpredictable and cruel. Within days of finishing the antibiotics, Meaghan's health began to deteriorate once again, and she developed pneumonia a second time. The oncologist was on vacation, and the doctor covering for him was not going to order the drugs because she felt that Meaghan did not have pneumonia. She felt that Meaghan's lungs filling with fluid was "part of the process." I refused to take no for an answer and told the Edmarc nurse that I didn't give a damn what the doctor thought, Meaghan was to get the drugs. If it meant that I had to take her to a local emergency room to get them, I would do it. I also told her to tell the doctor that even if it was disease progression, I had to look myself in the mirror every day for the rest of my life, and I wanted to make sure that I did everything in my power to save my daughter.

The nurse relayed my message, and the doctor ordered the medication. Meaghan was prescribed the same drugs that she had taken two weeks earlier. Her lungs did not clear quickly, but she did show signs of improvement. In retrospect, I agree that the doctor was correct in her assumption that Meaghan's pneumonia was disease progression, but faced with the same scenario, I would still demand the drugs.

The antibiotics slowly began to work, and by the weekend Meaghan had perked up and wanted to eat for the first time in days. Her favorite food was chocolate cupcakes, and Jim gave her one that had blue icing on it. Meaghan thought it would be hilarious to smear the icing on her lips, lie still in bed, and have Jim call me into her room to see if I freaked out!

He thought the joke was a little cruel, so he gave me a heads up and then called me to come to Meaghan's room. When I came into her room, Meaghan was lying completely still pretending to be dead. She had a silly smirk on her face and was literally biting her lips to stop herself from laughing. I tried to ignore her prank, but all she could do was howl with laughter. I was so happy to see her eating. Her spirits were high, and her cheeks were pink. The boys came home for the weekend, and we all hung out in Meaghan's bedroom, played games, and watched movies.

On Sunday evening, the boys returned to school, and Jim returned to Miami. They were all hesitant to leave, but Meaghan assured them that she was fine. I shared in their uncertainty, but we had all learned that in order to survive the abnormal, we had to follow a normal routine.

A few days later, the oncologist came to our house to check on Meaghan. Meaghan was alert, but her condition had changed drastically within the last twenty-four hours. The oncologist asked to speak to me privately. He suggested that I stop nursing Meaghan and consider "letting her go." I looked at him through my tears and said, "Absolutely not, and if this was your child you would do the same thing." The conversation was painful and austere. I was not convinced that this was the end. We had walked this path many times before, and I was certain that Meaghan would beat this setback one more time. He then asked to see Meaghan privately and soon afterward he and his staff left. I asked Meaghan what they talked about, but she said that the conversation was private and then changed the subject. This was completely out of character for her because she shared everything with me. Then Meaghan looked at me and said with a sigh, "All is forgiven; he tried, but he couldn't heal me."

That evening, Meaghan was weak but alert. She talked on the phone with Jim, as she did every night, and told him that she was fine and that he need not worry about her. She told him that she loved him but she was extremely tired and was going to bed early. Within a few hours her breathing became extremely labored and the "rattle" in her chest intensified. I immediately called Edmarc for advice. The nurse told me that she should be there within the hour to assess the situation.

By the time the nurse arrived, Meaghan's condition had worsened, and she began to drift in and out of consciousness. At times, Meaghan would interject a remark into the conversation, but for the most part she was silent, and her eyes were closed. Around midnight, Meaghan became quite talkative and asked me to drive her to Grafton High School. I assumed she was having a dream, so I agreed, but when I asked her why she wanted to go to the high school, her answer stunned me. She said that she wanted to tell her friends good-bye and hug them one last time. She mentioned several of her closest friends by name and thanked them for not abandoning her.

Meaghan then asked me to drive her home. Since she seemed to be having a dream, I suggested that she drive. She then opened her eyes, looked at me and said, "Duh, I don't have a driver's license" and closed her eyes once again. A few minutes later I told her that we were home, and she asked if the firemen were at the house to bring her inside because she was too weak to get out of the car. I replied, "Yes, they are." She smiled, thanked the fireman for helping her, and then I told her she was safely in her bed.

Meaghan appeared to fall asleep, but within minutes she became agitated and tried to pull herself into a sitting position. She opened her eyes and asked, "Is it February twenty-second, yet?" (As you may recall, she was not going to die before Jim's birthday on the twenty-first). I answered, "Yes."

Meaghan's Story

Meaghan then looked at me and said, "I'm ready to go home now." I replied, "You are home." She opened her eyes and said, "No, Mom I'm ready to go Home, but I'm paralyzed. Can you help me?" I replied "Yes. I'll get your wheelchair and I'll push you. Will that help?" I went into the hallway and brought the wheelchair into her room and placed it next to the bed where she could see it. Once she saw the wheelchair, the panic on her face disappeared, and she became relaxed. She then smiled at me and said, "Thank you, Mom, for helping me. I Love you."

Meaghan began to describe the journey she was taking and said that we were in a line with other people. She told me to slowly push her and said that she would direct me where to go. Meaghan described the others in line with her - people of every age, race, creed, and economic background. She told me that we were to enter a building and that she needed to get a ticket to go inside. I asked her where we were to go to get the ticket and she replied, "The girl with the cute pajama pants on has them. She will give us one, just keep pushing."

Meaghan described the building as rather ordinary. It had a long hallway with many doors. I asked her if we were to go through one of the doors and she said, "No, we continue going straight." She then reminded me that she would let me know where we were going and said to continue to push her. I asked her once again where we were going and she replied, "Home." A few minutes passed, and Meaghan opened her eyes and smiled the most radiant smile I had ever seen and said, "We turn at the Light" and then she yelled, "Papa!!" Just then, she elbowed me, and I fell out of her bed. I believe that that was the moment her spirit separated itself from this world.

Meaghan continued to describe where she was and said that she was on a beautiful white sand beach with Jim's dad and that the ocean was the most magnificent blue. She said he was healthy and that she and Papa were walking in the surf. She said Jim's dad had on a white polo, blue swim trunks, sandals, and a white baseball cap. She said she was no longer in her pajamas, but was wearing a bikini, tank top, and shorts. Being a sixteen-year-old girl, she then complained that she didn't have the proper shoes with her, and said that I really should have gotten her new flip-flops!

Over the next forty-five minutes, Meaghan became less verbal but continued to smile and laugh. When I asked her what she was laughing about, she replied that, "Papa was telling her jokes and explaining things." I was lying at the edge of her bed holding her as she described the journey that she was embarking upon. I realized afterward that it was one last gift that Meaghan was giving us all. She was letting us know that she was okay, affirming that there is indeed life after death and it's full of love and totally amazing.

By morning, Meaghan had stopped interacting with us. Unlike the previous times, she did not return to consciousness. I called both Jim and the boys and asked them to come home. Although she did not want them there to see her die, I felt it was necessary for them. Meaghan's spirit was gone; only her body remained. Our three dogs' sixth sense seemed to be in overdrive that day. They were agitated and wouldn't leave Meaghan's side. In order to get some needed peace and have some alone time with their sister, the boys and I decided to give them beer to calm their nerves. We had been told that this worked on a neighbor's dog during thunderstorms. It did work; the dogs calmed down and crashed next to Meaghan's bed. I think we may have given the puppy a little too much because when she awoke she appeared to have the "spins."

The Edmarc nurses never left Meaghan's side and told us that Meaghan could be in this "limbo" for hours, days, or even weeks, as there is no way of knowing what the body will do. Friends, teachers, and coaches sat with Meaghan and held her hand throughout the day. When each one left, they knew that the end would be soon. Jim arrived home later that evening. I told the Edmarc nurse that I was comfortable with the situation and that we would all take turns all night and would call if things changed. I felt that Jim needed alone time with Meaghan to say his goodbyes. I had my time, and I felt strongly that he needed closure as well.

Around ten that evening, Jim insisted that I go to bed. He said that he and the boys would stay with Meaghan. Since I had not slept in three days and was totally exhausted, I reluctantly agreed. I set my alarm for midnight in order to give Meaghan her medication. When I awoke I found her sleeping peacefully. There was no change in her condition. I administered the IV drugs, kissed her forehead, and then returned to bed. I still cannot explain what happened next.

Around 3:15, I heard a voice in my head say, "Get up. Don't go back to sleep." I walked to Meaghan's room where Jim was asleep. Meaghan's breathing had changed considerably in the last three hours. I told Jim to go to bed and that I would take over. I then got Meaghan's medications together, returned to her room, and whispered in her ear, "Mommy's here." Meaghan gave me a faint smile and then she took her last breath. I truly believe that she was waiting for me to return.

Completely stunned and somewhat unsure of what had just transpired, I called Jim and the boys to come to Meaghan's room immediately. TJ frantically began taking Meaghan's blood pressure, and each time he got an error code. The four of us stood silently in Meaghan's

Meaghan's Story

room looking at one another, completely dumbfounded by what we were witnessing. I'm not sure for how long we stood there. No one spoke – there was nothing left to say. For two years, Meaghan had fought with all her will. Like my sister and so many others, the world of reality crashed down upon us, and Meaghan, too, became a statistic. I then left Jim and the boys to stay with her and called Edmarc and told them that Meaghan had passed away peacefully in her sleep.

Chapter 12 – The Aftermath

Our world of hope ended at 3:42 AM, April 10, 2008, almost two years to the day after the initial diagnosis. Even though I had played this moment over in my head numerous times, there was a part of me that never believed that this moment would actually come. I was stunned and completely unprepared for the emotional and mental journey that our family was about to embark upon.

The Edmarc nurse arrived about half an hour after I called. She examined Meaghan, "pronounced," and then called the funeral home. Meaghan had been in a nightgown, but I knew she would prefer to be dressed in something more fashionable, so, with the nurse's help, I dressed her in her favorite sweats. The funeral home staff arrived within the hour. The nurse met with them, and they went to get Meaghan. The hall to Meaghan's room is short and zigzagged, so it was not possible to get the stretcher into Meaghan's room. Jim picked her up and carried her to the stretcher. We all kissed her goodbye. Jim told them to take good care of her... then we all broke down and sobbed.

Afterward, we called our families to tell them the terrible news. My first call was to my parents. As the phone was ringing, I kept praying that no one would pick up. Just as I was going to hang up, my mother answered the telephone. I told her that Meaghan had died peacefully in her sleep during the night, but my words failed to register with her. She kept repeating, "What are you telling me, what are you saying?" I told her again and again and again that Meaghan had passed away overnight. Eventually my mother said, "Oh, My God... I'll call your brother and sister." I don't think her reaction was due to her dementia; I think she was in shock.

As a mentioned before, both Jim and I had not been overly forthcoming to our aging parents regarding Meaghan's condition. We felt that it would be too much for them to bear. My parents had outlived two of their own children and now their youngest grandchild. It was an unbelievably cruel twist of fate. I told my mom that because of her declining health I did not expect her to make the trip. She replied that she would be coming and then began to sob. Jim called his family and then went to break the news to our village – the twenty-first century way – through emails and a post on Meaghan's Caringbridge site which read:

> *Our beloved Meaghan went Home this morning. She fought the disease for two years. It laid waste to her body while at the same time it brought forth a spirit and strength which left all that knew her in awe. She grew from gawky teenager to a beautiful, self-assured young woman who left us beaming with pride. She*

remains a symbol of courage to her family and friends and will be sorely missed. Her next journey will be one of peace and love. She's with her relatives in Heaven and will live forever in our hearts and minds. Her funeral preparations are incomplete as of now. We expect the service to be Monday evening but we will post details as they become available. Thanks to all for your kind words, prayers and friendship. Meaghan and the Herrity family will always remember the many kind acts.

Peace, Jim, Jan, Jimmy and TJ Herrity

> *"But they that wait upon the LORD shall renew their strength; They shall mount up with wings as eagles; they shall run, and not be weary; and they shall walk and not faint." Isaiah 40:31*

Jim and I showered and waited for the funeral director to arrive so we could pick a casket and make preparations for Meaghan's burial. He brought a book with caskets for us to look through. The choices were endless, and some even had themes. We chose the one that looked the most stylish and quickly closed the book. I think it took us less than five minutes to make our decision, as the process was just so surreal.

We then chose the cemetery and bought four plots from a private owner. Jim told the funeral director that they were for Meaghan, himself, me, and of course my next husband. It was tasteless but funny, and we all had a good laugh. The funeral director left and then our parish priest, youth minister, and choir director came to the house to discuss the funeral. As our priest began to discuss his preparations, I cut him off mid-sentence and pulled out a piece of paper from my pocket with my thoughts on what I wanted for her service.

Several months earlier I had planned every detail of Meaghan's service and hoped that I would never have to use that piece of paper. I wanted each song and Bible reading to be meaningful and reflect on the extraordinary young woman that Meaghan had become. However, I still wanted her service to be youthful. I was afraid that Jim and I would not be thinking straight and let her final sacrament in the Catholic Church be thrown together hastily because of our grief.

Jim and I then went off to the mall to purchase a dress and shoes for Meaghan to be buried in. Because she had been unable to walk in heels since this nightmare began, and due to her intense love of shoes,

Meaghan's Story

we decided that she would get a pair of sexy stilettos and new earrings to accessorize her outfit. We dropped the clothing off at the funeral home and then went home and literally collapsed.

Meaghan passed away during Easter break, and many of her friends were away visiting colleges. Several of her closest girl friends were on a trip to Italy, so we decided to have the funeral service on Monday evening and the burial on Tuesday morning, so they could also have closure. Before any of the girls' parents had the chance to break the news of Meaghan's passing, one of the girls on the trip received a text with news of Meaghan's death and details of her funeral. Several of the girls called home hysterically, begging their parents to spend thousands of dollars in airfare to bring them home for Meaghan's funeral.

The information we had received about their arrival time from Europe was incorrect, and the girls, including Meaghan's best friend, would not be back in time for her funeral service. The "lucky" teacher chaperoning the trip began working on a plan to cut the trip short for the girls and get them home on Sunday with minimal cost and disruption. I cannot even imagine how she dealt with twelve emotionally distraught teenage girls half way around the world who were determined to get home.

When Jim and I found out about the madness that was ensuing with her friends, we decided to add a second service/memorial just for the girls, to let them laugh and celebrate their friendship one last time. Our challenge was to find a restaurant in a nice location for a least a hundred people. Thank goodness for Google because our search provided the perfect location for Meaghan's celebration. I called late on Friday night, and luckily the banquet manager answered the phone and said that a room had just become available. There had been a cancellation within the last hour.

The banquet manger said that the room overlooked the York River and had views of the Chesapeake Bay. Meaghan loved the water, and the atmosphere was just what she would have chosen for her "send off." I told them that we would be right up and asked them to hold the room. After we signed the contract, both Jim and I agreed that finding this venue was more than a coincidence - If we had learned of the girls' dilemma earlier in the day, the room would not have been available. We both felt that Meaghan was still involved in her favorite pastime – spending money. I then called one of her friend's parents and told them of our plan and asked them to relay the message that Meaghan would want them to stay in Italy and enjoy the trip.

The following day, we had an appointment at the cemetery. We needed to pay a few of the expenses and sign papers to transfer the deeds to the plots into our name. A cemetery employee took us on a tour of the memorial park. We assumed that he was going to take us to our plots, but to our surprise, he began a sales pitch and tried to get us to cancel our earlier transaction and purchase plots in a more desirable area of the cemetery. This is a very distasteful side of the business, but it does exist. Because of it, we learned Lesson XXII: Death is big business, and it is the employee's job to make money for the cemetery or funeral home. The sales pitch can result in the buyer making an emotional purchase instead of a rational decision and spend money that they do not have because they are vulnerable due to their guilt or grief.

Once I realized what the salesman was doing, I demanded that he turn the car around and return us to the office. Once inside, Jim went to finalize the paperwork, and I went into the ladies room and began to sob. While I sat on the floor and wept, the paper towel dispenser started shooting out towels. To my amazement, it wasn't an automated dispenser. It was like someone or something was offering me a tissue to wipe away my tears.

After Jim finished the paperwork and we left, I asked him if he knew what the employee's agenda was on our tour. He replied, "Yes." I then asked why he didn't stop him, and he replied that he wasn't sure what I wanted. If I wanted to spend thousands of dollars more on the "gated community" as opposed to our "ghetto site," he wasn't going to stop me. I told him that I was fine with the location and about what had just happened to me inside the ladies room. Jim looked at me with tears in his eyes and said, "She was always very helpful."

We then had to go to the funeral home and see Meaghan. I wanted to make sure that her make-up and hair were age appropriate and that they did not make her look like an old lady. We called ahead, and they had her ready for us. Seeing her in a coffin was the most unbearable and surreal experience in both our lives. I adjusted her make-up and hair, and we placed personal items inside the coffin, kissed her, and left. We told the funeral director what had just happened at the cemetery and he said that he wasn't surprised – it's a dirty little secret in the industry. He said that was the reason he didn't have us order a marker. He wanted us to take our time to ensure that we did not overspend and regret the decision later. We then came home and prepared for out of town guests and I wrote her eulogy.

Meaghan's Story

Meaghan Colleen Herrity
September 6, 1991 – April 10, 2008

How do you sum up a life in five minutes or less? Meaghan was here only sixteen short years, yet left a mark that most of us do not achieve in the average seventy years of life here on Earth. Hers was a life of strength, courage, determination, humor, grace, endless love, and faith. She touched everyone she knew, and many she had never met. Her impact was huge and will reverberate for many, many years to come.

In the Broadway play Rent, the song Seasons of Love, breaks down the life of one of the characters in increments of time. The message is simply… time is precious, but often we think about time only when someone is ill. The message of the song is to live and experience life, make your journey meaningful, leave a legacy. Meaghan did just that. She got what her purpose was, she got what we are here on Earth to do, and her life was and IS a testament to that message. Her smile was thousand-watt, her sense of humor irreverent, her faith immeasurable, and she made all those around her comfortable. People loved her, and she touched many lives. When she became ill, her friends were put at ease by her smile and sense of humor. She never pitied herself, and carried on bravely, as if she only had a cold. When they came to visit, laughter filled the house. It was never an uneasy situation, never awkward.

Meaghan entered this earth on her own terms and left it the same way. She never met a challenge that dampened her spirit. She overcame obstacles with grace, courage, and with her sense of humor and personality intact. When she was told as a toddler that she was a big girl now and would no longer have a bottle, she did what all toddlers do. Yelled, "FINE," pushed a fax machine off our desk, and stomped out of the room, never to touch a bottle again. In seventh grade, Meaghan's nerves got the best of her, and she did not make the field hockey team. She came home devastated, listed her grievances loudly, and then went outside and started hitting balls. By the eighth grade, she became confident of her ability, strong, and then made the team with ease.

When her diagnosis came, facing a life threatening operation and told she would most likely die and definitely never walk again, Meaghan told us she could handle any treatment, fought the effects of the operation on her spine and then set out to work on walking again. Within months, she was taking steps and within a year, she was climbing stairs to her room. When the disease recurred and took her steps away, Meaghan simply started again, never to be beaten. Throughout the course of the disease, Meaghan insisted on being told the truth, no matter how scary, no matter how bleak. The decisions to never stop fighting the cancer were always hers. Faced with chemotherapy and side effects that ripped her body, she took the drugs without complaint.

In the two years following diagnosis, Meaghan was in constant pain; however she filled her days with school, friends, and laughter. Her courage and spirit touched doctors, nurses, physical therapists, friends, and strangers alike. When she finally decided that using a website would be a good way to share her journey, it inspired not only those who knew her, but many she had never met. That same spirit of never giving up served her well when the second recurrence came. Told that she would most likely die, and there was no longer a treatment option, the news only made her fight harder.

Don Samuels, her teacher, and field hockey coach, asked her friends to share their thoughts for the York County Courage Award.

Her best friend, Katie, wrote: Meaghan Herrity became the personification of courage on April 14, 2006. However, she has surpassed my definition of bravery and continues to do so every day. Meaghan has achieved more outside of school than most students attempt when they have the luxury of taking the classes inside of one. For her junior year, she currently holds an outstanding 3.8 GPA, keeps up with regular homework assignments, quizzes and tests, and is a member of the Grafton yearbook staff. This year Meaghan was almost unanimously chosen as Grafton's Junior Homecoming Princess and she stays in social circulation through her Facebook website, phone calls, instant messaging, and ceaseless visits from friends when she is in good enough health. Miserable as she felt, it is very rare to hear a complaint from Meaghan. What you can find in place of complaints is her incredible sense of humor and wit that bring smiles and laughter to whoever she comes in contact with. What I find most courageous about Meaghan Herrity is her ability to be optimistic in every situation that is thrown at her. Although cancer may have damaged Meaghan physically, it is certain that this obstacle has only highlighted the heroic qualities in her.

Her friend Shelby wrote: She started a charity in our school to raise funds and collect donations that will bring joy and comfort to other cancer patients going through rigorous treatment.

Meaghan's Story

Charlie wrote: Meaghan Herrity has been a friend of mine since elementary school. During freshman year, Meaghan was given dreadful news. She had been diagnosed with cancer. Two years later, she never lost her good humor or fun personality. In fact, one of the only things she had lost is her passion for ketchup.

Rachel wrote: Throughout the exhausting process of rehabilitation and chemotherapy, Meaghan has remained uplifting and an inspiration to all. She has homework spread out and bags from a shopping trip with her mom in the corner. She still has the concerns of a teenager. Although some would expect to find her in a depressed state, Meags always had a grin on her face and greets everyone with a huge smile. Within seconds, her optimism puts visitors at ease.

Taylor wrote: I've come to associate courage, as well as optimism and strength, with one of my best friends, Meaghan Herrity. After being diagnosed with cancer and given only six or more months to live, a normal 14 year old girl would have absolutely broken down. However, Meaghan's response was just the opposite. She continued to live her life as normally as possible and face her condition head on by getting every possible treatment.

We are honored and privileged that we were chosen to be Meaghan's family, to share her time on Earth with us, to love her, and we will forever hold her memory deep in our hearts. Her beloved brother, TJ, a young man of few words, summed her up by a simple phrase, "She was something." Our purpose here on Earth is very simple. We are here to make ripples. Meaghan made waves.

Chapter 13 – Resuming Life

During the weeks and months after Meaghan's death, much changed for our family, and each of us dealt with the tragedy in our own way. Early on, our combined grief felt like the proverbial "800 pound Gorilla in the room." I tried to help both the boys and Jim, but ultimately I needed to help myself first. Our grief counselor compared the grief process to the words used by flight attendants during the safety lesson prior to takeoff: "You need to put your own oxygen mask first before helping those around you." Essentially, I needed to heal myself first before I could help anyone else.

The grief process isn't easy, and it is a process. I read books on grief, books on the after-life, books on near-death experiences – anything that could give me a definitive answer to why this happened and what happens after you die. I read Socrates and Einstein, two of the world's greatest thinkers, hoping they could explain why a loving God could allow children to suffer, only to realize that they didn't have any answers either.

What I did learn was that grief is a powerful emotion. I had to confront my pain and sorrow in order to regain control of my life. This may seem like an easy task, but it took endless amounts of energy, hard work, and introspection to understand what had just unfolded in our lives. I came to the realization that I was experiencing post-traumatic stress syndrome. Although I wasn't technically a "combat veteran," I had been at war for two years and needed to acknowledge how Meaghan's illness and death had begun to influence every choice in my life.

I simultaneously struggled with anger and depression and dealt with my sadness by avoiding living. I passed on social gatherings, stayed close to home, ate way too many complex carbohydrates, and slept the day away trying to keep from feeling the intense pain. Then one day I realized that although the pain of losing a child was excruciating, it was the loss of Meaghan's future and her potential that was unbearable. That day a piece of my heart began to heal.

When I did venture out, I found the world a very different place. I had my first "break down" at the grocery store in front of the cupcake display a few weeks after Meaghan died. Cupcakes were Meaghan's favorite food, and no trip to the grocery store was complete without stocking up on the marshmallow filled delicacies. As I passed by the display, I reached to grab a few packages, and it hit me – Meaghan was dead. I didn't need to buy them any longer. I stood in the aisle with tears streaming down my face, trying to breathe, completely helpless, and filled with horror. I was so out of control that I panicked and left my semi-full cart in front of the display and drove home. To this day, whenever I am at a grocery store, I avoid the cupcake aisle, because it is yet another reminder that Meaghan is no longer with us.

For several months after Meaghan's death, I always wore sunglasses when I ran errands because I didn't want to be recognized. When I ran into people I knew, I could see the pity on their faces and the look of relief that it was my child that had died and not theirs. Most people would awkwardly express their sympathy, but I often ended up comforting them. It was a bizarre twist of fate.

Another thing that surprised me when I ventured out into the world was the number of exasperated parents I saw yelling at their children. Often a mother or father would strike the child to get them to behave. I always wanted to let the parent know how lucky they were that their child was walking, talking, and alive. But I said nothing - it is just another life lesson from losing a child.

One day I ran into a woman whom I was not particularly fond of in the grocery store. She saw me and turned away, startled. I was so sick of people being uncomfortable around me because of Meaghan's death that I literally chased after her and rammed my cart into hers, in essence turning the tables. It felt empowering. I said hello and engaged her in a polite conversation and actually felt like my old self for the first time in months!

I had told Meaghan that in time we would be okay, and I intended to keep my promise to her. I began to focus on the "To Do List" she had given me, but I was completely unprepared for the amount of energy that it would require. So, I began with the easiest thing on Meaghan's list – buying a Mercedes. Next, I took all of her field hockey t-shirts and t-shirts that were from special times in her life like dance recitals, summer camps, and family vacations and had a quilt made celebrating her life. I then created the Meaghan C. Herrity Charitable Foundation. Its mission is to provide a scholarship in Meaghan's memory each year at Grafton High School, to help other families struggling with pediatric cancer, and to lend financial support to the charities that were important to Meaghan and had helped us during her illness - especially Edmarc.

Meaghan asked me to thank all the doctors, nurses, and therapists that had helped her along the way. She and I had both come to respect and admire those who work in this field. The work that these individuals do each day is truly remarkable, and their ability to treat and minister to both the patient and the families is nothing short of miraculous. Lastly, Meaghan asked me to write this book and tell the world about who she was, how she lived, the challenges she faced, her sense of purpose, and lastly, that she was more than just data in a medical journal.

Meaghan's Story

Since I am not an author, I had no idea how to go about the process, so I began to write down my thoughts and read my journals. I was completely unsure of what I should say, and I had no idea if I could finish this book, let alone get it published. I felt that if I wrote it, I would be keeping my promise to Meaghan. Also, one day, my grandchildren could know about their amazing aunt and hopefully tell their children and so on and so on. Ironically, by reliving the "hell of her illness," I began to see the beauty in living, and I began to deal effectively with my grief. I had to give myself permission to be happy once again because I felt that enjoying life meant that I was being disloyal to my daughter. I still struggle with that daily, and I suppose I will for the rest of my life.

I know that this may seem odd, but there are days when I think I may have dreamed Meaghan's illness and death. It still doesn't seem real. Outliving a child is never in one's life plan, and the shock of it still reverberates with me daily. I know that acceptance is the final stage of grief, but I am not there yet and may never be. I do know I will never fully accept Meaghan's death, but as a family, we are learning to adjust to our "new normal." I have found that birthdays, anniversaries, and holidays are incredibly hard emotionally. Because of this, we have found a way to include Meaghan in our celebrations; We toast her on her birthday and add an extra place setting at the table to include her in our holiday meals. Erin included Meaghan in her wedding by placing a card at each table that read, "In lieu of favors, a donation has been sent to St. Baldrick's Foundation in memory of Meaghan Colleen Herrity."

Perhaps the most common fear of a bereaved parent is that others will forget about your child with time. We have been fortunate that Meaghan's friends continue to remember her. Each year on the anniversary of her passing, they release balloons at Yorktown Beach in her memory. This year we released sixteen green balloons for the years that Meaghan was with us and two white balloons for the number of years she has been gone. They also continue to write to her on her Facebook page, but she has yet to write back…

To acknowledge her absence at the last field hockey game of what would have been Meaghan's senior year, the varsity coach left Meaghan's position open for the first five minutes of the game and hung her jersey on the fence alongside the other senior girls. I could not contain my emotions as I was so touched by the gesture. After the game I was presented Meaghan's roses, which I then drove to the cemetery and placed on her grave.

Meaghan's high school planted a tree in her memory and dedicated the yearbook to her. She was also remembered by her classmates at their Baccalaureate and Graduation ceremonies. The athletic department created the Meaghan Herrity Courage Award to recognize a student athlete who has demonstrated remarkable courage on or off the field. The award is given at the year-end sports banquet, and the students who have received it are deeply honored to be chosen.

I walked alongside Meaghan during her illness but was often so busy wearing others hats (teacher, nurse, advocate) that the Mom role was not always front and center. I regret that. While writing this book I came to the realization that although I was Meaghan's mother, she taught me more about living and handling adversity than I could have ever taught her. Her inner strength and grace continue to inspire me, and each day I marvel at how she handled the twists and turns of her illness without anger or bitterness.

Meaghan's illness and death changed me as a person. I have found a calm and peace that I did not have before. Her description of the afterlife was a life changing moment and an enduring gift that changed me profoundly and permanently. I continue to experience moments in which I feel Meaghan's presence, and I am keenly aware that love and life do not end with death. I take comfort knowing that Meaghan's journey touched countless lives and that her life's voyage can be measured both in its richness and quality, as opposed to quantity of years. I learned the most important lesson of all through our journey – Lesson XXIII: Life and love are the greatest gifts we can give one another, and each day should be filled with kindness, joy, love, gratitude, forgiveness, and service to others.

Perhaps the most profound lesson of all was spoken by both my sister Karen and Meaghan in their final days. Both said that our journey here on Earth is all about loving each other and both said the following words: Lesson XXIV: It's so simple… it's all about love.

Meaghan's English teacher read one of her poems at what would have been her high school graduation ceremony and spoke these words:

"Meaghan Herrity was an exceptional student. She was also an exceptional teacher. She taught us how to live with hope and optimism. She taught us how to laugh with microwave peeps and sling shot monkeys. She taught us how to love – unconditionally and with forgiveness - and she taught us how to die – with grace and dignity."

I had finished this book when I came across what seemed to be a message from the great beyond on Meaghan's computer a few days before Christmas 2009. We purchased Meaghan a new computer in January 2008. She passed away in April of that same year. Her computer sat virtually untouched in her room for over a year until I began using it in the summer of 2009 when mine broke. Meaghan kept her iTunes on the computer. Since she had quite an extensive collection of Christmas

Meaghan's Story

music, I thought I'd create a playlist on my iPod and listen to some of her favorites to help me get in the mood for the holiday.

While pulling songs over to my iPod, I began to notice that many of the songs were played on December 24, 2008 (iTunes date & time stamps the last time a song was played), which seemed quite improbable because we were in Key West during that time period, and Meaghan's computer was in her room in Yorktown. I called Jim and the boys and asked them to take a look at what I was witnessing. They, too, were dumbfounded. Jim then noticed that it was not just Christmas songs that had been played, but an eclectic group of songs – many of them Meaghan's favorites. Many of the song titles let us know that Meaghan was still around, just not in "3D." I know it seems impossible, but it did occur. Listed below are the songs that played for a twelve-hour period, December 23 – 24, 2008. You be the judge.

	Name	Artist	Album	Last Played
1	The Only Difference Between Martyrdom and Suicide Is Press Coverage	Panic! At The Disco	A Fever You Can't Sweat Out	12/23/08 9:04 PM
2	London Beckoned Songs About Money Written By Machines	Panic! At The Disco	A Fever You Can't Sweat Out	12/23/08 9:07 PM
3	I Write Sins Not Tragedies	Panic! At The Disco	A Fever You Can't Sweat Out	12/23/08 9:11 PM
4	If You're Gone	Matchbox Twenty	Mad Season	12/23/08 9:19 PM
5	Jude Law and a Semester Abroad	Brand New	Your Favorite Weapon	12/23/08 9:23 PM
6	Somewhere Over the Rainbow	Katharine McPhee	Somewhere Over the Rainbow / My Destiny - Single	12/23/08 9:26 PM
7	Numb / Encore	Jay-Z & Linkin Park	Collision Course - Numb / Encore - Exclusive	12/23/08 9:30 PM
8	Hope	Twista	Hope - Single	12/23/08 9:34 PM

Janice Herrity

9	Baby Girl (2nd Version) [Remix]	Sugarland	Baby Girl - Single	12/23/08 9:38 PM
10	Hey There Delilah	Plain White T's	Hey There Delilah - EP	12/23/08 9:42 PM
11	Let It Snow, Let It Snow, Let It Snow	Michael Bublé	Let It Snow! - EP	12/23/08 9:44 PM
12	Grown-Up Christmas List	Michael Bublé	Let It Snow! - EP	12/23/08 9:48 PM
13	I'll Be Home for Christmas	Michael Bublé	Let It Snow! - EP	12/23/08 9:52 PM
14	Tim McGraw	Taylor Swift	Taylor Swift	12/23/08 9:55 PM
15	Teardrops On My Guitar	Taylor Swift	Taylor Swift	12/23/08 9:59 PM
16	Sing for the Moment	Eminem	The Eminem Show	12/23/08 10:05 PM
17	You and Me	Lifehouse	Lifehouse	12/23/08 10:08 PM
18	Waiting On the World to Change	John Mayer	Waiting On the World to Change - Single	12/23/08 10:11 PM
19	Hate It or Love It	The Game & 50 Cent	The Documentary (Edited Version)	12/23/08 10:23 PM
20	Misery Business	Paramore	Riot!	12/23/08 10:26 PM
21	Stupid Girls	Pink	I'm Not Dead	12/23/08 10:30 PM
22	Who Knew	P!nk	I'm Not Dead	12/23/08 10:33 PM
23	Long Way to Happy	P!nk	I'm Not Dead	12/23/08 10:37 PM
24	Nobody Knows	P!nk	I'm Not Dead	12/23/08 10:41 PM
25	I'm Not Dead	P!nk	I'm Not Dead	12/23/08 10:49 PM
26	'Cuz I Can	P!nk	I'm Not Dead	12/23/08 10:53 PM

Meaghan's Story

27	*Leave Me Alone (I'm Lonely)*	P!nk	I'm Not Dead	12/23/08 10:56 PM
28	*U + Ur Hand*	P!nk	I'm Not Dead	12/23/08 11:00 PM
29	*Runaway*	P!nk	I'm Not Dead	12/23/08 11:04 PM
30	*The One That Got Away*	P!nk	I'm Not Dead	12/23/08 11:09 PM
31	*I Got Money Now*	P!nk	I'm Not Dead	12/23/08 11:13 PM
32	*Conversations With My 13 Year Old Self*	P!nk	I'm Not Dead	12/23/08 11:17 PM
33	*Hidden Track*	P!nk	I'm Not Dead	12/23/08 11:21 PM
34	*Over and Over (Explicit)*	Nelly featuring Tim McGraw	Sweatsuit (Explicit Version)	12/23/08 11:25 PM
35	*The First Cut Is the Deepest*	Sheryl Crow	The First Cut Is the Deepest - Single	12/23/08 11:29 PM
36	*Boston*	Augustana	All the Stars and Boulevards	12/23/08 11:33 PM
37	*Missing You (Album Version)*	Tyler Hilton	One Tree Hill Volume 2 - Friends With Benefit	12/23/08 11:36 PM
38	*Fallen*	Sarah McLachlan	Afterglow	12/23/08 11:54 PM
39	*A Lifetime*	Better Than Ezra	Before the Robots	12/24/08 12:00 AM
40	*Track 03*			12/24/08 12:03 AM
41	*Ain't No Other Man*	Christina Aguilera	Ain't No Other Man - Single	12/24/08 12:07 AM
42	*Can You Feel the Love Tonight? (from the Lion King)*	Earl Rose	Color, Rhythm and Magic	12/24/08 12:13 AM
43	*Over It*	Katharine McPhee	Katharine McPhee	12/24/08 12:16 AM

Janice Herrity

44	*Tiny Dancer*	Elton John	Elton John: The Greatest Hits 1970-2002	12/24/08 12:23 AM
45	*Happy Xmas (War Is Over)*	John Lennon	The John Lennon Collection	12/24/08 12:30 AM
46	*Imagine*	John Lennon	The John Lennon Collection	12/24/08 12:33 AM
47	*Beverly Hills*	Weezer	Beverly Hills - Single	12/24/08 12:36 AM
48	*Bless the Broken Road*	Rascal Flatts	Feels Like Today	12/24/08 12:40 AM
49	*Where the Colors Don't Go*	Sam Phillips	Cruel Inventions	12/24/08 12:43 AM
50	*The Mixed Tape*	Jack's Mannequin	Everything In Transit	12/24/08 12:54 AM
51	*Bruised*	Jack's Mannequin	Everything In Transit	12/24/08 12:58 AM
52	*Dark Blue*	Jack's Mannequin	Everything In Transit	12/24/08 1:02 AM
53	*Kill the Messenger*	Jack's Mannequin	Everything In Transit	12/24/08 1:06 AM
54	*White Rabbit*	Jefferson Airplane	The Essential Jefferson Airplane	12/24/08 1:12 AM
55	*Wait for You*	Elliott Yamin	Elliott Yamin	12/24/08 1:17 AM
56	*Stay With You*	Goo Goo Dolls	Let Love In	12/24/08 1:20 AM
57	*Let Love In*	Goo Goo Dolls	Let Love In	12/24/08 1:26 AM
58	*Sailing*	'N Sync	'N Sync	12/24/08 2:12 AM
59	*Giddy Up*	'N Sync	'N Sync	12/24/08 2:16 AM
60	*It's Not Over*	Daughtry	Daughtry (Bonus Track)	12/24/08 2:19 AM
61	*Leave the Pieces*	The Wreckers	Stand Still, Look Pretty	12/24/08 2:27 AM

Meaghan's Story

62	*Have a Nice Day*	Bon Jovi	Have a Nice Day	12/24/08 2:31 AM
63	*I Want to Be Loved*	Bon Jovi	Have a Nice Day	12/24/08 2:35 AM
64	*Welcome to Wherever You Are*	Bon Jovi	Have a Nice Day	12/24/08 2:39 AM
65	*Who Says You Can't Go Home*	Bon Jovi	Have a Nice Day	12/24/08 2:43 AM
66	*Last Man Standing*	Bon Jovi	Have a Nice Day	12/24/08 2:48 AM
67	*Bells of Freedom*	Bon Jovi	Have a Nice Day	12/24/08 2:53 AM
68	*Wildflower*	Bon Jovi	Have a Nice Day	12/24/08 2:57 AM
69	*Last Cigarette*	Bon Jovi	Have a Nice Day	12/24/08 3:01 AM
70	*I Am*	Bon Jovi	Have a Nice Day	12/24/08 3:05 AM
71	*Complicated*	Bon Jovi	Have a Nice Day	12/24/08 3:08 AM
72	*Novocaine*	Bon Jovi	Have a Nice Day	12/24/08 3:13 AM
73	*Story of My Life*	Bon Jovi	Have a Nice Day	12/24/08 3:17 AM
74	*Who Says You Can't Go Home (Featuring Jennifer Nettles)*	Bon Jovi & Jennifer Nettles	Have a Nice Day	12/24/08 3:21 AM
75	*Breakaway*	Kelly Clarkson	Breakaway	12/24/08 3:25 AM
76	*Since U Been Gone*	Kelly Clarkson	Breakaway	12/24/08 3:28 AM
77	*Behind These Hazel Eyes*	Kelly Clarkson	Breakaway	12/24/08 3:31 AM
78	*Walk Away*	Kelly Clarkson	Breakaway	12/24/08 3:38 AM
79	*Don't Cry Out Loud*	Melissa Manchester	Don't Cry Out Loud	12/24/08 3:42 AM

Janice Herrity

80	*Before He Cheats*	Carrie Underwood	Some Hearts	12/24/08 4:04 AM
81	*Making Memories of Us*	Keith Urban	Be Here	12/24/08 4:08 AM
82	*Be My Escape*	Relient K	Mmhmm	12/24/08 4:12 AM
83	*Who I Am Hates Who I've Been*	Relient K	Mmhmm	12/24/08 4:16 AM
84	*Hands Down*	Dashboard Confessional	Hands Down - Single	12/24/08 4:19 AM
85	*Deja Vu (Featuring Jay-Z)*	Beyoncé featuring Jay-Z	Deja Vu - Single	12/24/08 4:31 AM
86	*Ordinary Miracle*	Sarah McLachlan	Charlotte's Web (Music from the Motion Picture)	12/24/08 4:34 AM
87	*Mr. Brightside*	The Killers	Hot Fuss	12/24/08 4:38 AM
88	*Cool*	Gwen Stefani	Love, Angel, Music, Baby	12/24/08 4:45 AM
89	*Can You Feel the Love Tonight?*	Elton John	One Night Only	12/24/08 4:49 AM
90	*Pretty Girl (The Way)*	Sugarcult	Start Static	12/24/08 4:56 AM
91	*Track 10*			12/24/08 5:01 AM
92	*Karn Evil 9: 1st Impression, Pt. 2*	Emerson, Lake & Palmer	Brain Salad Surgery	12/24/08 5:06 AM
93	*Photograph*	Nickelback	Photograph - Single	12/24/08 5:10 AM
94	*If You're Reading This*	Tim McGraw	Let It Go	12/24/08 5:15 AM
95	*O Holy Night*	Céline Dion	These Are Special Times	12/24/08 5:20 AM
96	*Write You a Song*	Plain White T's	Every Second Counts	12/24/08 5:24 AM
97	*Somewhere Over the Rainbow*	Judy Garland		12/24/08 5:27 AM

Meaghan's Story

98	*Goodbye for Now*	P.O.D.	Testify	12/24/08 5:31 AM
99	*Better Days*	Goo Goo Dolls	Better Days - Single	12/24/08 5:35 AM
100	*How The Grinch Stole Christmas*	Jim Carey		12/24/08 5:41 AM
101	*Such Great Heights*	The Postal Service	Give Up	12/24/08 5:45 AM
102	*Stay Away*	The Honorary Title	The Road Mix: One Tree Hill, Vol. 3	12/24/08 5:50 AM
103	*You'll Ask for Me*	Tyler Hilton	The Road Mix: One Tree Hill, Vol. 3	12/24/08 5:54 AM
104	*Lay Me Down*	The Wreckers	The Road Mix: One Tree Hill, Vol. 3	12/24/08 5:57 AM
105	*Non-Believer*	La Rocca	The Road Mix: One Tree Hill, Vol. 3	12/24/08 6:02 AM
106	*We Do This to Ourselves*	Sherwood	Sing, But Keep Going	12/24/08 6:09 AM
107	*The Town That You Live In*	Sherwood	Sing, But Keep Going	12/24/08 6:12 AM
108	*The Sweet Escape*	Gwen Stefani	The Sweet Escape	12/24/08 6:16 AM
109	*Swingin' On a Star (vocal: Frank Sinatra)*	Tommy Dorsey & His Orchestra	Sentimental Swing	12/24/08 6:19 AM
110	*(More Bounce In) California*	SOULKID #1	Americanized	12/24/08 6:23 AM
111	*Let It Snow, Let It Snow, Let It Snow*	Harry Connick, Jr.	When My Heart Finds Christmas	12/24/08 6:25 AM
112	*Santa Claus Is Comin' To Town [Live]*	Bruce Springsteen	My Hometown (Single)	12/24/08 6:39 AM
113	*Someday*	Nickelback	The Long Road	12/24/08 6:42 AM

Janice Herrity

114	*Not Ready to Make Nice*	Dixie Chicks		12/24/08 6:46 AM
115	*Drops of Jupiter*	Train	Drops of Jupiter	12/24/08 6:54 AM
116	*Drops of Jupiter*	Train	Drops of Jupiter	12/24/08 6:59 AM
117	*What If You*	Joshua Radin	Catch and Release (Music from the Motion Picture)	12/24/08 7:03 AM
118	*As I Am [Intro]*	Alicia Keys	As I Am	12/24/08 7:05 AM
119	*Go Ahead*	Alicia Keys	As I Am	12/24/08 7:10 AM
120	*Superwoman*	Alicia Keys	As I Am	12/24/08 7:14 AM
121	*No One*	Alicia Keys	As I Am	12/24/08 7:18 AM
122	*Like You'll Never See Me Again*	Alicia Keys	As I Am	12/24/08 7:24 AM
123	*Lesson Learned*	Alicia Keys Feat. John Mayer	As I Am	12/24/08 7:28 AM
124	*Wreckless Love*	Alicia Keys	As I Am	12/24/08 7:32 AM
125	*The Thing About Love*	Alicia Keys	As I Am	12/24/08 7:36 AM
126	*Teenage Love Affair*	Alicia Keys	As I Am	12/24/08 7:39 AM
127	*I Need You*	Alicia Keys	As I Am	12/24/08 7:44 AM
128	*Where Do We Go From Here*	Alicia Keys	As I Am	12/24/08 7:48 AM
129	*Prelude To A Kiss*	Alicia Keys	As I Am	12/24/08 7:50 AM
130	*Tell You Something (Nana's Reprise)*	Alicia Keys	As I Am	12/24/08 7:55 AM
131	*Sure Looks Good To Me*	Alicia Keys	As I Am	12/24/08 7:59 AM

132	*Bye Bye Bye*	*NSYNC	No Strings Attached	12/24/08 8:03 AM
133	*This I Promise You*	*NSYNC	No Strings Attached	12/24/08 8:07 AM
134	*No Strings Attached*	*NSYNC	No Strings Attached	12/24/08 8:11 AM
135	*That's When I'll Stop Loving You*	*NSYNC	No Strings Attached	12/24/08 8:16 AM
136	*I Thought She Knew*	*NSYNC	No Strings Attached	12/24/08 8:19 AM
137	*Collide*	Howie Day	Stop All the World Now	12/24/08 8:23 AM
138	*Silent Night*	Sarah McLachlan	Wintersong	12/24/08 8:27 AM
139	*My Band*	Eminem	D12 World	12/24/08 8:32 AM
140	*Ay, Ay, Ay*	Karyme Lozano	Ay, Ay, Ay - Canción de la Semana	12/24/08 8:37 AM
141	*Track 01*			12/24/08 8:42 AM
142	*Pennies From Heaven*	Louis Prima	Elf: Music From The Motion Picture	12/24/08 8:44 AM
143	*Sleigh Ride*	Ella Fitzgerald	Elf: Music From The Motion Picture	12/24/08 8:47 AM
144	*Let It Snow, Let It Snow, Let It Snow*	Lena Horne	Elf: Music From The Motion Picture	12/24/08 8:49 AM
145	*Far More*	The Honorary Title	Scream and Light Up the Sky	12/24/08 8:54 AM
146	*O Holy Night*	Emmy Rossum	Carol of the Bells - EP	12/24/08 9:02 AM
147	*It's All Coming Back to Me Now*	Céline Dion	Falling Into You	12/24/08 9:10 AM
148	*Because You Loved Me*	Celine Dion	Falling Into You	12/24/08 9:14 AM

Chapter 14 – The Men in Meaghan's Life Speak

What I learned on Meaghan's journey – Jim, her Dad

When asked to make a contribution to this book, I thought it would be an easy task, but it turned out to be nearly impossible. As a father, I always felt that my role was to try to protect my family, especially my children, and solve whatever problem was at hand. However, unlike fixing a broken toy, or opening my wallet for a special purchase that was vetoed by Jan, I could not fix what was broken inside Meaghan, and I felt as though I had failed her.

GLIOBLASTOMA was a word that I had never heard in my life. Upon receiving the definition, it surpassed all other words that symbolized evil, horror, despair, and agony that I would ever use again. Hearing it for the first time, as a diagnosis for a condition that my precious daughter had, was the equivalent of getting the heart punch of all time.

There are some very beautiful people on this planet. Nurses, doctors, staff people who care for the sick out of something beyond a belief in money and security. These are the people that the definition of a calling is just that. Something that you cannot simply put a tag on but it merely is. Meaghan was blessed to meet many of these people in her journey, such as her Brooke, Teresa, Becky, "Herbie," and countless others.

We met the clergy, both local and from far away, who gave evidence to a divinity not present in sermons or tabernacles. Priests from our local church visited Meaghan frequently, as did the lay staff. None had or could offer any explanation as to why she was chosen for her burden. Monks from the Bronx's St. Bernard Monastery appeared when Meaghan was in her hospital one day and comforted her with their presence. They visited and showed compassion for the sick out of no reason than that was what they do. As mentioned, a Buddhist monk from Korea showed up unexpectedly next door and helped Meaghan with his acupuncture and healing herbs. His appearance was a strange coincidence but greatly appreciated and welcome. We have friends of all faiths, each sending prayers to their God for her healing.

There are also an incredible amount of really apathetic, horrible people populating this planet. People who think it's more important that they jump into an elevator ahead of a young girl in a wheelchair because the two minutes they might gain in being a complete jerk will make a difference in their so called lives. People who felt that anything inconveniencing them, such as a teenage girl pushing her in a wheelchair in front of them on the sidewalk, was an obstacle to be surmounted even if it meant pushing the young girl to the side and making her feel invisible.

We met people in the healthcare profession (never nurses or doctors) but the support staff that have many people in their midst who don't understand what a calling is, and wouldn't if you spent a year explaining it to them. This happened twice during Meaghan's journey, once when these individuals felt it was completely proper to have a barbeque chicken meal at 3:00am in the morning, complete with accompanying loud laughter and high pitched squeals of delight. And when confronted by parents, they at the time looked at us as Martians who bring messages beyond their understanding. This happened a second time while Meaghan was shopping in a hospital gift shop. One of the hospital employees stepped over her legs as they sat in the legs rests of her wheelchair, to grab an item on sale. There is no way to correct inappropriate behavior but perhaps me mentioning it the book will make the administration of hospitals more aware and council their employees on compassion, empathy, and etiquette.

There are many people in the world who are suffering – whether it is from famine, poverty, war, or just the sickness in your family. While this is a personal crisis, most people, for no other reason than a goodness in the human spirit, step forward to take just a little of the burden off of you. Friends were tripping over themselves to help us move into a new home while we were away in Boston with Meaghan. Craftsmen could not do enough for us in making the house accessible to Meaghan when she did arrive home. They took many extra steps that made her life easier, for no other reason than they could see this happening to them. Friends lessened the load for the couple of years with visits, food, and just showing the caring. It was a wonderful eye opening to my jaded soul.

When trying to understand what was happening to Meaghan and what I could do about it, I spent nights on the web going to bulletin boards, websites, and other resources to learn what we were fighting. I found many other people who were fighting or who had fought and lost but were continuing to help others to beat the monster of cancer. Many great suggestions came from people who were known only by their first name, but wanted to help. The list of angels, in this case, the children dying from glioblastomia, continued to climb during the two years of the battle. The parents of the angels in many cases continued their fight in the hope that they could help prevent the cancer from taking another. There are many beautiful people out there and it does smack of divinity.

Angels do exist on the earth. People who taught us that the hospice was not a dead end, pick up the pieces, nice to know you type of

Meaghan's Story

thing but rather people full of love and laughter for their patients. People who would come out in the wee hours of the morning from an hour away without a single thought. People who were there for you when something had gone wrong in the day and would sit there just because they might be needed. The angels from Edmarc Hospice are people that I will never forget to thank as long as I have breath.

The amazing curative powers of a street vendor's sausage hoagie is another blessed discovery. When running Meaghan around downtown Boston in a wheelchair, over the lovely cobblestone streets and non-existent sidewalk ramps, Meaghan was nauseous and looking pretty green. Due to the treatments she was receiving, she could barely eat some days and this day was no different. Passing a street vendor and taking a whiff of the sausage hoagies covered with onions and peppers, Meaghan thought a hoagie might be the thing for her. Wondering about the effects on her delicate stomach and potential germ content, we said what the heck? Meaghan ordered a large hoagie with everything and made short work of it. Color was in her face and she was the happiest she had felt in a while.

I am a traveling consultant so I was gone four days out of the week, which was excruciating to leave my daughter, but nonetheless I had to keep working. Most of the day to day care fell upon my wife, except on weekends. I would try to telecommute as often as possible and thankfully my employer was very compassionate about our situation. When home I would accompany Meaghan and Jan to chemotherapy. I was always amazed that they were somewhat desensitized by the oncology clinic. I suppose it became second nature to them. I never got used to seeing the amount of children with cancer. I never could figure out why it wasn't the lead story on every news program in the country.

However, there is courage in all people. The question is – when will it emerge? Does courage in a game, full of rules, officials, time limits and protective gear equal courage? How about hearing a word such as Glioblastomia as a fourteen year old and trying to understand what this means to your happiness? You must now decide if you are going to allow this word, as horrible as it is, to shape the rest of your life or whether you will seize life and make it shine. Meaghan had the choice at that point of curling up into a ball and hiding for the rest of her life. The choice she took of taking life into her hands, determining that she was going to fight until her last breath, was one that will leave me in awe forever.

Meaghan took her destiny unto herself, with bravery and a single mindedness to win despite the odds. She was told following her surgery that she would never walk again. Through sheer ferociousness of spirit, she was walking in the months that followed. Her determination at Physical Therapy was astounding to me, having seen her sometimes passive and distracted at field hockey. When she had to put every ounce of her being into getting up and walking, she showed all the courage of a commando. There was no longer the complaining young lady at practice but rather a determined woman who would not fail. It is amazing the blossoming that occurred in a few short months.

In choosing to live her life on her terms and not the cancer's terms, Meaghan was always surrounded by friends, books, music, and love. She voraciously read and listened to music as if she wanted to learn everything there was to learn at a breakneck speed. That she also included volumes of teen trash and chick flicks to accompany the classic novels she devoured was also part of the wonder that was Meaghan.

I've heard someone say that angels will be born to people and live some of their lives with us, leaving when it was time. To say Meaghan was an angel is not farfetched, but she could be a devil as well. My first encounter with Meaghan upon emerging from the womb was to be handled this blue eyed, mess of wet hair who owned me within a second of making eye contact. The angelic aura disappeared quickly when the nurse informed me I was to hold Meaghan until Janice had some additional work in another operating room. I was given specific instructions – I was not to feed the little lady. Meaghan proceeded to chew me out for the next two hours, while never losing eye contact with me. The look of 'how stupid are you' was one I learned very well over the years. When a nurse finally had pity on me and allowed me to feed her, the look was replaced with the 'Good Daddy, I hope you know who is in charge' and a look that I would see countless times again over the next sixteen years.

But regarding the angels living among us, I'll take that as a comfort that Meaghan was something special. One day she was a teenage girl thinking that N'Sync was the most important thing on the planet. The next day she discovered that life and living it well was what it was all about. She took every day as the next best day of her life. She laughed with her friends, cried with her best ones, never showing the world the fear that was in her, but only displayed a happy visage for all to see. As chemicals wracked her body, she took each treatment without complaint and looked at the next one as something that would allow her to beat the disease within her.

She showed me how to live my life and that is something I will never forget. Her two years of hell were also two glorious years of taking every second together as a gift and allowing us to imprint her love and courage into our hearts forever.

Meaghan's Story

From Jimmy – Meaghan's Oldest Brother

What can I say about my sister that hasn't already been said in excruciating detail? I could say I miss her, but that would be redundant and an understatement. I obviously do miss her and I think about her daily. But I can honestly say I don't often reminisce to times after she got sick, it is just too hard. I've really tried to block it all out and not think about any of it. So, I guess this is therapeutic to discuss how her illness and death have affected me.

I was almost six, and proudly enrolled in kindergarten, when Meaghan was born. That being said there was definitely a gap in our ages, and thus it effected how we interacted with one another. We weren't necessarily close growing up, but we were still brother and sister and definitely loved each other. How did we express our love? Like most siblings, we fought... but nevertheless, we always had each other's back.

When Meaghan became ill, it struck us all unexpectedly. She had complained about back pains the day before and went to the emergency room to be examined, but they found nothing unusual. The day that our world changed was just an ordinary day. I went to class and then to work. Meaghan was acting dramatic all week, which was not uncommon, so her being taken in the ambulance that morning did not weigh heavily on my mind. I just assumed she was being a teenage drama queen. Only when my mother came running into the house, covered in her own vomit did it register that something was terribly wrong. My mom told my brother and me the events that were unfolding at the hospital and I remember just being in shock. I knew that I needed to assist in any way I could.

After Meaghan was diagnosed with cancer and was told that she would never walk again; I remember feeling numb. Meaghan was always so healthy it all seemed like a bad dream. What amazed me most was that Meaghan ignored the doctor's predictions and refused to accept what would be most people's norm, and live her life as a paraplegic. She fought daily to regain the losses from the cancer and, despite all the doctors' expectations, she managed to walk again. This miraculous recovery was not to last, and she had a relapse, and once again lost the ability to walk. That was absolutely heartbreaking to witness ... but she was not broken and she was resolute in the fact that she would beat both the cancer and paralysis again. I, too, believed she would beat both – I never thought otherwise.

I don't remember much of what I did during her illness. My parents insisted that we continue with school and our lives and truly hid much of Meaghan's illness from us. But, I tried to be both emotionally and physically available to both my parents and Meaghan. I would go with my mom to the hospital, therapist, or anywhere else when she needed help with Meaghan.

Meaghan and I shared a common interest in books, music, and movies. I cannot recount all the times during her illness that I would go out on Tuesday night for the newest book or movie that was released at midnight. It was something I could do for her. Although small, it made me feel like I was helping. She had eclectic taste in books, from Jane Austen to Gossip Girls, and she introduced me to the Harry Potter books and DVD's to which I am very grateful. She loved music and her taste ranged from the Irish Tenors to Rap. When she became ill, she exposed me to a lot of music that I may not have liked otherwise. I credit her with introducing me to Fountains of Wayne, and the Killers. When I hear both of those bands I always think of her....

When Meaghan's illness became progressively worse and she became bed ridden, I would hang out in her room – watch movies, listen to music, or play board games with her. What was most amazing was that she was always positive and never complained about her illness. She had an amazing inner strength and an amazing inner light. I truly always believed she would beat her illness and am still shocked that she did not. Our collective hope got us through her illness.

What I learned from my sister and her illness is this. You can't predict life and you must participate fully in it each day, It is vital that you be emotionally, mentally, physically and spiritually present for your loved ones… because life can change or end without warning.

From TJ – Meaghan's Other Brother

Meaghan was my sister and her experiences, and the whole ordeal itself, did have a profound impact on me. I can easily say that most of my journey was of a spiritual, emotional, intellectual, and philosophical nature. What transpired was quite real, and perhaps so very real that even now there are short interludes in which I forget it ever even happened.

Suddenly there I am, walking away from the ice cream store on Yorktown's Riverwalk with my mother and sister, summer treats in hand and my mother commenting on how overpriced that ice cream is. Now the scene changes and it is me and my sister, perhaps one or two of her friends in tow, together in my derelict red Ford Contour and stopping by the 7 Eleven on our way home from track practice purchasing some of those delightful, and addicting Slurpees. Until finally reality snaps me back to the present, and I emerge from my dream. It would be a terrible lie if I were to say there were not times when I do wish that I could return

Meaghan's Story

to a simpler, more pleasant, and innocent time in my life. I know that is not the case, and what was cannot and never will be again, and shall not be in the future with such outings with Meaghan, which is a luxury many other sets of siblings have. These memories, especially the common and unremarkable ones, I must keep close to my heart and treasure forever, for there will be no more.

The best place to begin the rest of this tale is at the very beginning – April 14, 2006, the day my mother came screaming into the house uttering news that would change my world forever.

April 14, 2006 for me began when I was awakened before my usual time of 5:45 in the morning from the screaming of my sister fighting with my parents. They had insisted she get over herself and go to school that day, as she had stayed home several days due to back pains. Knowing her, none of us at the time thought it was anything more than a teenage girl drama in overdrive. So after a short scene at the top of the stairs, I got ready, left the house, and caught the bus. It was such a typical day that I remember no details of between the time I left the house and the time I returned that afternoon. I walked through the door and began to unpack when after one or two minutes my mother burst through the front door telling me that my sister had tumors in her spine. This came to me as quite a shock so I went upstairs to my room to do an internet search in order to find out more.

I discovered that there were three types of spinal tumors: outside of the spinal cord , inside the spinal bone, and inside the spinal cord. Being a natural optimist and knowing that according to my research tumors on the outside of the bone were the most common, I came to the assumption that was what she had. It was only a few hours later that I received a phone call from my parents confirming my worst fear – the tumor was inside of the spinal cord, and we learned later on in her journey that there were multiple growths.

In the months following Meaghan's diagnosis, I began to try to figure out what caused her cancer and I came to the conclusion that we would never know. The human body and its systems are so complex and when something that complex is thrown out of order, only chaos can come. That is what cancer is. It is unchecked cell growth and mutation, and in the end could be triggered by one measly molecule falling out of line.

In the end, I suppose it all comes down to chance. Although some day science may be able to explain it, reason never will. It will always be baffling how a perfectly normal and healthy girl who was running miles around a track at the beginning of the week would be lying

in bed paralyzed due to a cancer inside her spinal cord five days later...
Luck can be a strange thing.

    About a week and a half before my sister's passing, I received a call one morning from my mother, with a hint of sobbing in her voice, informing me that my sister had fluid in both of her lungs and difficulty breathing. She was certain this was it. She was certain that this was the end. We had been down this road many times prior, almost always expecting what we most deeply feared, and what we knew was inevitable. Yet each time, after we had braced ourselves for the worst, we found ourselves relieved. My sister rebounded from whatever near-death experience she had and continued on. Although not one of us wished to believe it, we still prepared ourselves for the worst each time. We were grateful every time my sister recovered, but after countless of these experiences, the sudden relief became just as stressful as the news of my sister's deteriorating condition had.

    It is not an easy task preparing for the loss of a loved one, and neither is the discovery that the preparation had been in vain. It began to take a toll, and there was always an air of uncertainty surrounding my sister. Would she make it or would she not? If she began making long strides towards a recovery, would it last or would it suddenly come crashing down? It was an emotional rollercoaster.

    Yet somehow I knew that this time it was different. That this time it was really going to happen. While it is true that I had prepared myself, I know I do not have to explain that I wished what was about to happen did not have to come to pass. My brother arrived after a few minutes after my mother's phone call to pick me up to take me home. If we were lucky, we would make it just in time to say goodbye. Do understand that my brother's car, an old blue Ford Mustang, is absolutely disgusting. The interior of that car is littered with kinds of garbage that I had not known to exist. Yet it is this unclean and unholy place that I made the most unlikely cathedral. I prayed to God, or to whatever else is out there, truly for the first time in my life.

    Do not mistake me for your typical heathen. Like a good Catholic boy, I had always been sure to say my prayers before meals and before sleeping. I said everything from the classic Hail Mary to a simple "thanks for the food." It was all lip service, I never truly felt any connection to a God or Great Spirit in any of my prayers before. In fact, the most sincere I had ever been in praying prior to this had been my asking of God to make sure that either the Boston Red Sox or New England Patriots did not blow the game when all seemed right. I was never really a spiritual man.

Meaghan's Story

But on that day I did believe. On that day I did feel something. I asked whoever was out there for just a little more time to be with my sister. I did not expect an answer, and I even thought I was asking for a little too much, but I asked anyway. And I truly did feel some sort of connection, as if something out there was listening.

My brother and I made it home after a typical length trip. It had been about forty minutes since he had picked me up. As my moment of prayer had been quite brief, taking only a minute or two, I spent most of the ride in quiet thought. I wasted no time getting out of the car and through the front door. I had to get to my sister as quickly as possible. To my surprise, however, I was greeted by my mother with a relieved look on her face. She told me that Meaghan's lungs had just suddenly cleared up. It was a miracle, and I was in disbelief. So I ventured down the side hall to where she was. Meaghan was sitting up in bed, a big smile on her face. Since I had classes the next day, my mother hastened us out the door and sent us on our way. I was still in shock.

I would visit home that weekend, little knowing it would be the last one I would spend with my sister. It was just another weekend to me. I remember first heading to Best Buy in order check to see if they had the film *Serenity* in stock. That night I put the DVD into my laptop and began watching it. It was early in the morning, not yet light, and I was assigned with keeping watch on my sister while my parents slept. About an hour into the film, I heard Meaghan cry out to me, so I stopped the movie and went into her room. The birds were annoying her. She could not sleep they were so loud. I listened and I heard the birds outside, singing their morning song. It was not overly loud, but my sister's senses were so sensitive at that point even the slightest sounds were torture for her.

But she wanted me to stop the birds from singing. As much as I wanted to help, I knew it was impossible. I could not stop a force of nature. That is one of the few times in my life when I knew something was out of control and I understood that no course of action I took could provide any relief. I am not sure any analysis or commentary on faith, the nature of God, or religion can be drawn from this. It is really a rather ordinary and unremarkable incident, but it has been embedded in my memory and replayed rather often in my mind for just over two years. The only reason I can think of this being so important to me is the fact that this was the last time I spoke to my sister, because the next time I saw her she would be unconscious.

I received the call on a Wednesday afternoon. I was just leaving an English class when I was told I was needed at home immediately. I knew it was not good. Once again I was taken home by my brother, and I prayed again. This time it was different. I knew I would not be answered.

Janice Herrity

I knew that there would be no repeat of the miracle that had taken place the week before. The week before I had only asked for just a little more time. I still wonder today if I should have instead asked for a full recovery, but it does not matter. I knew then, riding in the car, that it was the end.

When I saw my sister in bed, unresponsive, I could not bear it much. I spent some time with her, whispering words, but I eventually retreated to my room where I fell asleep after awhile. I would be awakened by my mother early Thursday morning, only a few hours after midnight. My family then kept vigil. Around 3:40 am, my mother noticed that she had stopped breathing. Occasionally there would be a deep breath, and then nothing for minutes. The last time I felt a pulse from her was at 4:09 am. Then it was over.

I recall in the hours and days after her body was taken out of the house that a sort of energy lingered. It was most present in her room. While my mother and I are the only ones who seem to have felt it, I am without a doubt certain that something lingered. My mother said to me that after Meaghan died, I cited a rule of science stating that neither energy nor mass could be destroyed. I, of course, do not remember this, but I trust her word. Perhaps it may be pseudoscience but there could be some truth to those words. I cannot claim to know what happens after death, but I do know that I refuse to believe it is the end. The human mind and essence is a complicated thing.

Although that aura in my sister's room has long since dissipated, there are still events that I have been unable to explain rationally. Dreams, as real as they seem (almost as if messages from the departed), can be explained by the fact they are dreams. Shortly after my sister died and her room was being cleaned, a teddy bear mysteriously moved after people had left the room. No one had any idea who moved it, but they all claimed they did not. This could be taken as a sign that Meaghan was watching, or it could be explained by the senility of the cleaners. Strange things continued to happen for weeks after her death. One day two of my sister's friends stopped by and my mother took them into Meaghan's room sensing that they wanted to be near her. While in the midst of the conversation, my sister's pillows (which were battery operated) began to light up... no one was near them, they just spontaneously turned on. The first summer after Meaghan's death, almost every evening our dogs would awaken around three am and run excitingly through the hallways, barking as if they were chasing someone or something. Then the episodes ended as abruptly as they began, when I mentioned to my mother that it was strange that the dogs weren't barking in the middle of the night any longer. To my astonishment, she said that she told Meaghan to stop worrying about us, enjoy her new life and we would be okay and someday we'd all be together again.

Meaghan's Story

In regards to the "Spooky Play List" discussed in my mother's segment of the book, that I cannot explain rationally, as much as I would like to. I first assumed that the play times had been transferred to the computer when the iPod was synced to it, however, since the list had a running time of nearly ten hours, and late at night, it could not possibly have been my mother. She is not a late night person, and many of the songs are not ones she would have listened to. Under the impression that the computer somehow turned on and opened up iTunes, I looked for patterns in the songs played. There were none to be had after I sorted it under various categories. I found that sorting the artist, album, song title, genre, or any other category would not result in a continuous list. If that could not be done, all the songs being grouped together without a break, then it is not possible that iTunes being accidentally opened was the explanation. The list is too spontaneous and random for it to be explained by a random song in the library being set to play for ten hours until the computer shut down, and even then the computer would not take that long to turn off when unattended. Having ruled out what was impossible, I could only assume that this was deliberately done. The question is by whom?

I still do look for a logical and earthly explanation for the so called "Spooky Play List", and perhaps a reader of this book will offer one, but I still keep an open mind. I do not know what happens to us after death, but it is quite possible that as energy we can continue to interact with the world. In fact, many popular explanations for ghosts include energy interacting with electrical devices. There may be nothing for us after we depart this world, although I do not like to believe that. Nevertheless I find it to be an exercise in futility to try to fully comprehend what lies beyond because it is simply beyond our understanding, and the truth will not be known to us until our journey is over. So I choose not to worry. We must make the most of the short time we have, comforting ourselves with the knowledge that there is something greater for us at the end.

Chapter 15 – Meaghan Speaks

Once more the story I am about to tell you will seem hard to believe, but it is true. I had finished this book (or so I thought), when I stumbled upon these poems stored in Meaghan's desk. How I happened upon them is the hard to believe part. I talk with my daughter every day and always before I go to sleep at night. I told Meaghan one evening the book is all done, almost ready for print. I was just rereading it and doing some last minute edits. I said to Meaghan if there is anything you want added or deleted, let me know.

I fell asleep only to be awakened by a nagging urge to go into the attic and open Meaghan's top desk drawer. Once I did, I found the following four poems. The desk had sat in the attic for over three years, we never moved it downstairs with her because her new room was not large enough to accommodate all her furniture .

I then began to look through every other box that had her things stored in them, leaving the attic in complete disarray. I found nothing else. I then came downstairs and started searching all the word documents on her computer and came across a file that had two more poems. I do not know when Meaghan wrote them and all are untitled, but I can only assume that since they were in with her homebound school work it was when she was ill. I will let you, the reader, be the judge of what her message is…

Poem 1

Another night in suburbia
All the house lights now have been out for hours
It's the time of night
When the only souls awake
Are the scorned roaming the streets
The only light they see
Is the tip of their cigarette butts

No one would expect
A seemingly perfect young girl
To be wide awake
Looking in a hand mirror
And silently sobbing
When her reflection isn't what she wants
Even though others notice her
For her excellent personality
She can't stand being Miss Congeniality

Janice Herrity

All the she wants is to be called beautiful

There are so many forms of beauty
Internal beauty is a quality
That many see as important
For one who has external beauty
Is often cherished at a greater height
Than someone who lacks seemingly perfect features
And when a young girl cannot sleep
Because she wants to look like the faces in the magazines

Many look past external beauty
And look at internal beauty

Poem 2

You can't see the weakness in her
She hides it away from the world
So no one can see it but her
The world will watch her play a part
In which she has never been hurt
She's never cried

Poem 3

In the darkness of the night
She sits up, awaken by a nightmare
She hates the person she has become
Tears fall from her hand
And silent screams
Not meant to be heard by others
But only she can hear
Only she can see
Only she can feel this nightmare
Becoming her day to day reality

She wears long sleeves in summer
To hide the pain from others
Picture perfect on the outside
She may look golden
But all her emotions are stone
Only in the darkness of the night
Does this seemingly perfect girl let her golden fire melt to liquid
Why would this beautiful girl

Meaghan's Story

Degrade her self-esteem to an all-time low
When nothing is wrong

Poem 4

The night is dark
And she's all alone
Screaming soundlessly
Crying silently
Dying slowly
She's all alone
Nothings right
Everything s wrong

Nightmares of the future
Become the present
She's too skinny
She's too pale
And all she can do to fix it is cry
Slashing her wrists
Making her horror story
The past

She's lost in a world
Of swirling colors
Crying
Dying
The she wakes up
And realizes
Everything might go right
The nightmares are gone
Finally her eyes lose the red
And her arms are tan
She eats again
And she
breathes

Poem 5

The wail of sirens fills the air and cuts through quiet of the night
Flashing, whirling, red and white lights
Illuminate the dark as they rush to a frightening incident
And save a life, if the clock is still ticking

Janice Herrity

Behind the locked door is a horror show
From the other side all that can be heard is the sound of running water
Water that seeps beneath the door, tinted with red

In the hallway outside the locked bathroom door
A mother's screams for help echo, and two silent children
Wide-eyed and scared, huddle together as they cry
Afraid of what could be behind the door, and afraid
That there might be nothing left behind
Help finally arrives and storms the house

Poem 6

I sit alone on the shore
Lonely, without you
I hear your voice in the sea
Your spirit finds me
A wave washes over me

  I also came across the following which Meaghan wrote a few weeks before her death. it was an English assignment. I am not sure what the prompt was, but it was in preparation for a state writing assignment. She was very ill at the time, and she connected to a morphine pump for pain management. You can see the effects of the drug in her writing, as her thoughts often ramble. Her emotions are very raw and brutally honest. Meaghan rarely showed her vulnerability as she was trying to protect everyone around her, which is not unusual for many children who are facing death.

  Meaghan writes:

  For many years, decades and even centuries, those who are considered the brightest among us such as scientists, doctors, biologists, and philosophers have regularly asked themselves the same question. The question is why some people who have been healthy their entire lives and have good morals and don't drink or use drugs, don't get to live past a certain age and there is no cure for their terminal illness at all. The question is why some people who drink and do drugs have no health problems and why others who run and are active every day suddenly wake up not being able to walk.

  In the early weeks of April 2006, when I was in 9th grade and 14 years old, I started having weird dreams about

Meaghan's Story

people around me dying. In late March, I played in an indoor field hockey tournament where I played goalie. During the game I noticed an incredible pain on the left side of my neck. After one game the coaches put ice on it and I continued to play. The pain eventually went away. Two days later, I woke up and noticed I walked clumsily and couldn't turn my head. I thought I had the flu.

Eventually I went to the doctor and got pain killers for what they thought was a pinched nerve, but it became harder to walk. The next day I couldn't get downstairs because I was too weak. The next night I had nightmares and sweats. I went to the bathroom and couldn't stand up. An ambulance took me to the hospital where they did some tests and took me to CHKD. I had surgery two days later to remove a tumor from my spinal cord. An MRI later found two more tumors that the doctors couldn't see in the surgery because of the swelling. We went to Boston and I started radiation, chemotherapy, physical therapy, and occupational therapy.

I eventually learned to walk with and without crutches, but it all disappeared a year later when all the sudden I couldn't turn my head, or walk, or sit up… it was even worse than it had ever been. We went to Duke to start a medication regimen but I could only tolerate one of the medicines. The other one gave me blood clots. What I had learned physically started disappearing. I planned on returning to school this year, but I was too weak and couldn't sit up without throwing up.

Now I have pain all over. I have a morphine drip 24/7, steroids and other medicines for seizures that started randomly and for internal body shaking. I'm trying acupuncture and herbal treatments.

The question I would like answered is if there could be some kind of sign that there was something wrong with a kid. If there was some kind of test that would show a problem, they could start treatment earlier. If you could give a person another day in their life, no matter how old or young they are, they would have something to look forward to. Maybe treatment could start earlier and it wouldn't be so harsh, and the kids could live longer, and there wouldn't have to be a child who couldn't go out and play. They would not have such a bumpy road.

It's hard to watch kids who are used to being outside playing hooked up to tubes. It's hard to make a hospital room seem like a home. Why can't we identify something before it gets this

Janice Herrity

big? Why can't kids have a chance at a longer life and be able to go outside and play? Why do some people have a "Get Out of Jail Free" card and others have a "Do Not Pass Go" card?

Chapter 16 – Life Lessons Learned

Lesson I: Time is money and a hospital, even a children's hospital is a business.

Lesson II: As a parent, you have rights and can accompany your child or loved one anywhere in a hospital with the exception of the operating room.

Lesson III: Do not assume that a resident will be able to give you accurate information just because they are a doctor, wait for someone who has finished their training to inform you of tests results.

Lesson IV: Hospitals and insurance companies control just about everything in regard to treatment, and they expect a fair amount of compliance from the patient and the families in return.

Lesson V: We were not in control.

Lesson VI: When someone in the family is diagnosed with cancer, they do not get it alone, the whole family gets cancer.

Lesson VII: Always double check medications, as errors do occur within the medical community.

Lesson VIII: No one should face a hospital stay without a family member as a support system or as an advocate.

Lesson IX: Understand what you are signing when you enroll a loved one in a medical study and do ask questions. Do not feel pressured to sign anything until you are completely aware of what you are signing.

Lesson X: Inform the technicians or other hospital personnel of any limits or special circumstances regarding the patient. Do not assume they know everything about your case.

Lesson XI: Life is a Gift, live each day with joy in your heart. Love, laugh and forgive, as no one is promised a tomorrow.

Lesson XII: The world is not handicap accessible.

Lesson XIII: Anger is counter-productive

Lesson XIV: The outpatient world of a hospital operates much differently than the inpatient world. Procedures and equipment in an outpatient setting are geared for patients needing more intensive rehabilitation than in a hospital setting.

Lesson XV: Trusting your physician and being truthful are crucial to your treatment and success.

Janice Herrity

Lesson XVI: Within a short amount of time after an MRI is completed, the radiologist reviews the scan and then dictates the results on a recorder. Radiologists can determine quickly if there is an area of concern, especially if they have previous scans of the patient to compare with.

Lesson XVII: Call your local social service agency, especially in the case of a child and discuss your situation, they may be able to assist you.

Lesson XVIII: It is my belief when others give up on you, you give up on yourself. Friends are the best medicine of all.

Lesson XIX: Get a second opinion even if the news is good, because cancer has a tendency to "hide." It only takes one mutated cell to regenerate a tumor.

Lesson XX: The insurance company calling the patient and directing you to certain hospitals is for their benefit and to control their costs. They are a business and will direct you where it is beneficial for them.

Lesson XXI: It is Virginia law that if anyone passes away at home without a DNR (Do Not Resuscitate), your home becomes a crime scene. Family members are separated and interviewed, until a resolution by emergency personnel can be reached.

Lesson XXII: Death is big business, and it is the employee's job to make money for the cemetery or funeral home..

Lesson XXIII: Life and love are the greatest gifts we can give one another. Each day should be filled with kindness, joy, love, gratitude, forgiveness, and service to others.

Lesson XXIV: It's so simple ...it's all about Love.

About The Author

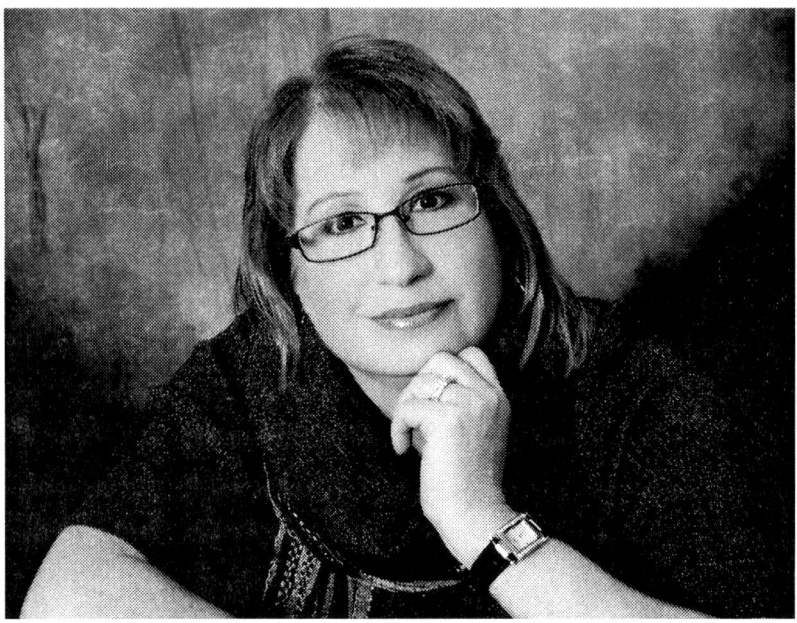

Janice Burnham Herrity was born and raised in Elmira Heights, New York. After graduating from Alfred State College in Alfred New York, she went to work for the Kmart Corporation as a management trainee and remained with the company for nine years, eventually becoming a District Manager. She is now the Vice President of Operations for the Herrity Group Inc.

After the birth of her second son, Janice decided to leave the rat race to become a stay at home mother, a decision which she has never regretted. She has been a tireless volunteer for countless community organizations throughout the last twenty-five years and is the president and founder of the Meaghan C. Herrity Charitable Foundation.

She wrote Meaghan' Story as a promise to her daughter and has rediscovered the love of writing she had in her youth.

Janice lives in Yorktown, VA with her husband Jim and two sons.

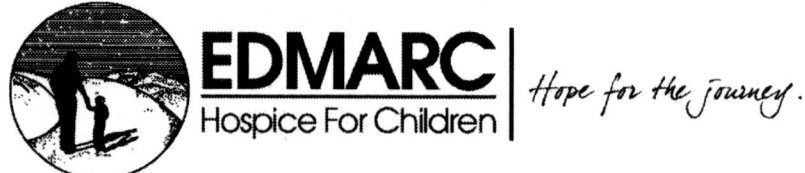

The mission of Edmarc Hospice for Children is to ease the trauma of a child's illness or death and to reduce the disabling effects of pediatric illness, loss and bereavement on families.

Edmarc was begun by members of Suffolk Presbyterian Church in Suffolk, Virginia in 1978. Edmarc was created by a minister who was dying of cancer and a young couple whose only son was dying of a progressive neuromuscular disease. The minister's name was Edward; the boy's name was Marcus. The agency is named in their memory.

Edmarc Hospice for Children was the first hospice in the nation designed specifically for children. Edmarc is the only pediatric hospice organization in Hampton Roads, Virginia. The mission of Edmarc Hospice for Children is to ease the trauma of a child's illness or death and to reduce the disabling effects of pediatric illness, loss, and bereavement on families. Edmarc's health care services allow a child with a life-limiting illness to stay at home whenever possible. Remaining at home helps alleviate some of the child's stress and can make healthcare for the child less traumatic.

But when a child is ill, Edmarc never forgets that the entire family is affected. Families who have a child with a life-limiting illness experience a high level of stress, including emotional, social, spiritual, and financial pressures. This stress often becomes debilitating to the entire family, sometimes resulting in dysfunctional family dynamics, financial hardship, and divorce. To help families cope, Edmarc offers a broad range of services to address not only the physical and emotional needs of the child, but the multi-dimensional needs of the family as well.

Edmarc's home health, hospice, and bereavement support services are available to children and families 24 hours a day, seven days a week. Since 1978, Edmarc's program has grown steadily, indicating a need for this unique type of care. Edmarc has served over 950 families in Hampton Roads and more than 3,300 family members in the past 31 years.

The out-of-pocket costs incurred by a family with a member who is catastrophically ill are enormous, regardless of the availability of health insurance. Frequently, when a little child is diagnosed with a catastrophic illness, one parent must leave their job to care for the ill child, or loses their job because of multiple absences from work, leaving a family that was dependent on two incomes to survive with more expenses on half the income. Our statistics show that Edmarc's intervention significantly decreases the family's financial burden by decreasing hospital days and increasing access to financial resources. Numerous published resources cite a divorce rate of 75% in families where a child has died. In Edmarc bereaved families, the marriage failure rate has been less than 20%. Because we serve a pediatric population and do not receive reimbursement through Medicare, we rely on philanthropic sources for nearly 90% of our budget.

If you are interested in knowing more about Edmarc or if you would like to contribute to Edmarc in some way – through direct gifts to the organization or through the purchase of other needed items for Edmarc families or by simply donating valuable time – please feel free to contact the organization at (757) 967-9251 or visit www.edmarc.org.